The
Conflict
of
Caring

~

*A loved one, a nurse, a patient
Finding the path to wellness from all sides
of the bedrail*

Judi Schofield, RN

The *Conflict* of *Caring*
A loved one, a nurse, a patient
Finding the path to wellness from all sides of the bedrail

www.judithschofield.com

ISBN: 1479146935
ISBN-13: 978-1479146932

Contents

To my husband Rob,
Who resides forever in my heart.

.

Introduction

Have you ever been sick and needed medical care? Has a loved one ever been hospitalized for an illness? Living through the experience of a serious medical diagnosis brings to light the effect illness has on the human perspective and the whole experience can be frustrating to say the least. Facing the fear of being sick is one thing, but trying to understand the system that is supposed to return us back to health and well-being is quite another.

Communication is the key to any successful relationship but it is especially true when we are sick. With millions of people being hospitalized each year, the chance of being in a medical situation is likely. At some point, the majority of the population will either be a patient or have a loved one who needs medical treatment, and how they perceive the care they receive is vital to the physical and emotional outcome of these stressful situations.

With the current attention on family centered care and the bombardment of information through technology, understanding the reality of illness and the array of human emotions connected to it is as important as the medical treatment we expect to receive. Illness is not just a physical situation; it is also an emotional one, and telling our story is a way to share our experiences and understand the perspectives from all sides of the bedrail. It is where science meets society and a new understanding of each is found.

This book is the story of my journey through the healthcare system from all three perspectives. Although it is a personal story, its appeal is universal. A husband in critical condition; becoming a nurse later in life; being diagnosed with cancer; all three experiences eventually leading to a place of understanding and healing after many bumps in the road. Hopefully through the sharing of my experiences, the gap in awareness between family, nurse and patient is narrowed and healing can begin.

Part One:

The Family View

"Lots of people want to ride with you in the limo, but what you want is someone who will take the bus with you when the limo breaks down."

— Oprah Winfrey

Chapter 1

Sick and Tired

I turned around as I reached the top of the hill, panting and wiping the sweat away with my sleeve.

"What's the matter, babe? Can't keep up with the old wife?" I laughed as I sat down on the curb to wait for him to catch up.

My husband was a little more than three years younger than me and anytime I could compete with him and win, I did. I watched as he struggled to walk up the last half of our street, and my laugh faded into concern.

"Are you alright?" I asked as I stood up and headed toward him. His face was pale, he struggled to breathe, and his face was soaking wet. He dashed ahead of me as I reached out to him, laughing, telling me he would beat me anyway he could.

He made it to the top of the street and we walked the rest of the way, but I could tell it took all he had just to make it home. Looking back now, it was the first indication that something just wasn't right.

It was the middle of a cold and dreary January, and we had made a New Year's resolution to lose weight. Rob and I went out for a walk every night but recently we had started to run a little bit. Neither one of us was very fast, but we would laugh and say we could get home quicker to eat a snack before going to bed.

This night was different, though. Even though he said he was just trying to win, I knew differently. Worry set in. And the last thing we needed was worry. Rob and I had experienced our share of hard knocks in the past, and we were looking forward to some better times together.

I looked at him from across the room as we ate our ice cream, laughing at our not-so-effective-diet. We had been married for six years and he still melted my heart. He was a handsome man, with dark black hair, an infectious smile, and beautiful steel green eyes that sparkled when he laughed.

Many times people would ask me how I got such a good-looking husband.

"What am I, chopped meat?" I would ask and laugh. But he looked different now. Pale, dark circles under his eyes; not the vivacious man I knew and loved.

A few nights later, those symptoms escalated.

"I am so sick", he said as he paced throughout the house. Please take me to the hospital."

As we headed toward the ER, I tried not to panic, but it was difficult. Rob never wanted anything to do with doctors, so when he asked to go to a hospital, I knew it couldn't be good. I had to drag him in just for routine checkups so this was out of the ordinary.

We arrived to find a packed waiting room. Friday nights are usually a busy time for emergency rooms and this one was no exception. Knowing patients get seen in order of need, I scanned the room and wondered where we fit in the mix. There were some on crutches and others sleeping curled up in the waiting room chairs.

I looked at him as I chattered away as I do when I am stressed; I either talk or eat, and food was not readily available. He looked horrible and I wasn't sure what I would do with him if he decided not to wait.

Rob had a stubborn streak and if he said "Let's go," nothing I could say would change his mind.

My throat was dry after four hours of useless conversation, but finally his name was called. "Thank goodness," I thought to myself.

After a short examination, it was determined that he needed to see a gastroenterologist, a stomach doctor, because of his vomiting and severe abdominal pain. But, because the emergency room was overflowing with patients who had what seemed like immediate needs, he was given a prescription and told to follow up with a specialist sometime over the next week.

"Can't you see how busy we are?" the doctor said as he pushed open the curtain that separated us from the next stretcher. These other patients are really sick and need attention now. You need a doctor's appointment, not an emergency room visit."

We looked at each other in amazement. There was nothing else to do but go home.

"I feel like a child being scolded for misbehaving," Rob said as we headed back to the car. He then proceeded to double over and vomit into the blue plastic basin that he was given on discharge.

Rob continued to get worse and within 24 hours, he was so short of breath, he could only sleep sitting upright.

I was a licensed practical nurse working in one of those urgent care centers, or "Doc-in-a-Box" as they were called. It wasn't my dream job but it did get me off the night shift, which I had worked for years.

I had Rob come down to see our physician, even though I knew he could not admit patients to the hospital. As he placed the stethoscope on Rob's chest, I could see the concern on his face.

Dr. Jack, as we called him, had a short stocky build and a sweet round face that squinted when he examined a patient. I had worked with him long enough to recognize the different facial expressions he made as he was determining his diagnosis and I did not like this one.

He did an EKG and told me that it was so abnormal, he could not accurately give us a diagnosis.

"I am not sure what it is, but he is a sick man," he said as he began to call the neighborhood doctors to find one who would take his case.

Many of the local physicians did not want to be associated with the urgent care center, but finally, after a lengthy conversation with Dr. Jack, one agreed to admit him as a patient.

After we packed him a bag and called his workplace, I drove Rob to the hospital, relieved that someone was finally going to help him. They quickly settled him in and said his doctor would be in later that night.

When I left him that evening, he said he felt a little better and would probably be released in a day or so. I gave him a quick kiss and headed home to take care of the kids.

The phone startled me, and it took a moment to realize what it was.

"We are moving your husband to the Intensive Care Unit (ICU) tonight," were the words that brought me to my feet. Before I could respond, I was assured that this was not serious.

"We want to give him some medication that needs closer monitoring," they explained. "There is nothing for you to do now. We just wanted to inform you of the transfer."

I was able to talk to him for a few minutes and he said he was okay and he would see me in the morning. I never closed my eyes the rest of the night. Medications for what? What the heck was going on?

As I arrived early the next day, I was met by two physicians and taken directly to a conference room. I had not worked in a hospital in quite a while, but I knew this was not the normal routine.

"Where is Rob?" My voice quivered. "I want to see him." Even though the door was closed, the noise from the ringing monitors in the ICU could be heard in the background and I worried it might be Rob.

"Your husband is seriously ill," they began. He has cardiomyopathy; his heart is very sick."

"His heart?" I asked, confused and upset. I stood up and leaned across the rectangular oak table. "Forty-eight hours ago your ER told us it was his stomach, reprimanded him for coming to the emergency room and then sent him home. Now you are saying it's his heart?"

I was angry but knew Rob's health was in their hands, so I had to remind myself to settle down and try to absorb the information.

They explained that they had nothing to do with the emergency room experience; that was in the past. All they knew this present day was that Rob's heart was failing fast.

He had something called cardiomyopathy and it was so severe, his liver was now extremely swollen. Something called congestive heart failure was the cause of all his vomiting and abdominal pain.

Dr. Carter, as he had introduced himself, continued with the diagnostic explanation but I couldn't take it all in. My head was swirling and for the next few minutes, his voice sounded like the Charlie Brown teacher on TV…"Wha, wha wha wha wha wha," is all that I heard.

Having to force myself to focus on their every word, I was finally able to ask, "What is his prognosis?" And for the next 20 minutes, they proceeded to tell me.

Even though I was a licensed practical nurse (LPN), I had no medical knowledge of cardiomyopathy. I had worked on an orthopedic floor and then the urgent care center, so I had no exposure to heart ailments. This disease was foreign to me.

I had heard the term a few years earlier when Rob's dad was sick, but never really understood it. I thought 54 years old was so very young when his dad had died at that age, but Rob was only 34. What was this disease that had a hold on my husband and our family?

I looked across the table at the two middle aged men. I wondered how many times they had sat with families and given them information that would affect the rest of their lives.

Did it still bother them? Was it just "another day at the office?" Had they ever been on the receiving end of medical information that affected their families?

The short gray haired man had a warm smile and he was the first to speak. He gave me the best explanation he could in the short time span we had together. The other one would nod his head in agreement but said nothing.

There were drugs that could manage the symptoms; they could "tune him up" for a while, but eventually, he would need a heart transplant.

"Heart transplant?!" I screamed out loud. My God, this was beginning to sound like science fiction to me. I fell back into my chair. The doctor who spoke took my hand while the other looked at his watch.

Their immediate prognosis was correct, and Rob did get better. He came home a few days later on some medications and quickly settled back into his normal routine. He didn't make a big deal out of it so neither did I, but the doctor's words were always in the back of my mind.

Rob was going to be followed by a cardiologist so I assumed everything was okay. At least for now. Every time I tried to bring up the subject of his health, he would smile and say he was fine. There was nothing else to do but to try to get back to normal, whatever that was.

Our lives had so many twists and turns before this diagnosis, but in comparison, that part of our lives looked good now.

Rob and I had re-connected at a neighborhood softball game several years earlier. Our families had known each other for many years, and we grew up just a few streets apart. My youngest sister and his were best friends and our mothers attended PTA together.

I always thought of him as "a kid" while growing up because of our age difference. When you are in school, three, almost four years is a big gap in age. He actually dated my younger sister for a while, so he had spent some time at our house.

Eventually, they broke up and all of us went our separate ways. I married and had a son while living in West Virginia, and Rob joined the

Navy. He married as well, but eventually both of us ended up divorced and moving back home.

One Sunday, I went to a local softball game to watch my sister pitch. Rob was on the other team, and, afterwards, we talked for hours. I invited him over for a cookout, and two years later, we were married.

There were many ups and downs during those two years, but we made it through, and a year later, we had another son, Adam. We were all a family now and looking forward to brighter days ahead.

Rob adored my son Jeff and vice versa. He coached his sports teams and took him camping with his friends. One time after they returned from a fishing trip, Jeff and his friend told me how much fun they had playing roller coaster in Rob's van.

It was an old VW van with paintings on the sides that reminded you of the 60's. If you opened up the back, you would expect to see peace signs and hear "Let the Sun Shine In" on an old 8 track player. It was left over from his "hippie" days, as he called them, and he loved that old vehicle almost as much as that time of his life.

I glanced at him from across the table as they continued with the story, and he was half laughing and half cringing as he shrugged his shoulders and tried to subdue his smile. The boys chuckled as they told how Rob would speed down the hills to gain enough momentum to make it up the next incline because the van had such little horsepower.

"Geronimo," they would yell on this roller coaster ride, and throw their arms up in the air as they sped down each hill.

As the story progressed, we all got the giggles and laughed all through dinner. That was the kind of father he was.

He hated the word "step parent." "Parenting is determined by actions, not blood," he would always say when people made comments about his close relationship with both Jeff and Adam.

His mom told me that when we first started dating, she worried because she thought maybe his interest in me was because of his affection for Jeff. He loved him so much, and she hoped he loved me as much as my son.

She said girls were always calling their house to talk to Rob, but he never showed much interest in them. Now, here he was married to a divorced girl who was older than him and had a child.

"I don't have to worry about that anymore," she said smiling and giving me a big hug. It made me feel good.

Rob was the type of guy that everyone liked; laid back, funny; not too much bothered him. I was more the "Type A" personality, worrying about pretty much everything.

I had been raised in an alcoholic home, so it was hard for me to break out of that pattern. His spirit was so contagious, though, I was beginning to lighten up.

"First you raise kids, and then you raise grass," he said to me one day when I was aggravated.

I had done some yard work earlier, and when I looked out the window, there he was playing soccer with Adam and a few of the neighborhood kids in that very spot where I had just gardened. I relaxed and went out to cheer them on. He had that kind of effect on me.

We were pretty much the typical family and we tried to return to some type of normalcy after his diagnosis. "The crazy side of normal," Rob would call it and we would all laugh.

The kids were doing well in school, Rob returned to work, and I got back into my running routine.

Jogging was something I enjoyed. I had run a few 5K races and Rob would sit and wait for me at the finish line. Afterwards, we would go get a bagel and a cup of tea. That time alone was precious to us, and we would sit and talk for hours.

He seemed to be dealing with his diagnosis pretty well and rarely even talked about it. Because he handled it so well, so did I, but I thought about it every day.

That November, I decided to try to run the local 10K Thanksgiving Day Race. Rob and I went the night before to pick up my packet because I was nervous about running that distance and wanted to be prepared in the morning. It was the compulsive side of me.

As we walked across the street that brisk night to get to the YMCA pre-registration site, I noticed he was short of breath. I rationalized that it was the cold weather, but the next day as I looked at him across the Thanksgiving Day table, he looked tired and pale.

He had slept in that day, missing my race. He was boasting to the relatives about my race time, but I really wasn't listening. The worry and concern was taking over again and I wasn't sure what to do. As I drove home that night, he slept in the car.

Over the next week, Rob's breathing became more labored. I knew he was sick when he went back to the emergency room for help.

"I have cardiomyopathy and I think I am in heart failure," he told the ER doctor.

Rob was the type of guy that learned all he could about the things he needed to know. Once he was diagnosed, he read and studied about this disease, and he knew as much about cardiomyopathy as any medically trained person.

It appeared they did not appreciate Rob diagnosing himself, because over the next hour, they did everything to prove he was wrong; chest x-ray, blood work, but not a cardiac work up.

The final diagnosis from the ER was bronchitis, and he was given a prescription for an antibiotic and sent home again.

For the next five days, I watched my husband move closer and closer to death. I would beg him to go the emergency room but he refused. "I will not be humiliated again," he said, gasping for each breath.

He could no longer lie down to sleep so he spent his time in a chair. He would cough and cough until he couldn't cough anymore, and then try to convince us he was okay.

When he would doze off for a few minutes and the coughing stopped, the kids and I would stand over him to make sure he was breathing; we were almost relieved when he coughed again.

I would call the cardiologist and leave messages and I always got an excuse—he was doing cardiac catheterizations that day, he was making rounds, he was seeing patients. I would leave a message but when they weren't returned, I'd call again. I ran back and forth—begging Rob and calling the doctor—to no avail.

Sometimes I would go out and just run and run; I was so frustrated and angry, scared and worried. The emotions were overwhelming and our lives were solely in the hands of the person answering the phone. Was I doing enough? Whom could I call? What should I do? Dear God, help me. What should I do?

Finally, at 7pm on a Tuesday evening, the cardiologist returned my call. I had an instant flashback of Shirley McClain in "Terms of Endearment" shouting as loud as she could, "Just get my daughter the medicine!!"

I suppressed the urge to scream into the phone, "You are supposed to be taking care of my husband!" Instead, I remained composed and told him how Rob was deteriorating and my frustrations with trying to reach him.

His only answer to me was that it sounded like Rob needed some medication adjustment.

"This happens sometimes. It's usually a minor tune up. Do you want me to admit him tonight or do you want to wait until morning?" he asked.

"I don't think he will live until the morning," I said with a cracked voice.

"Okay," he said to satisfy me. "I will call in some orders."

I immediately hung up and knew I now had to convince Rob he needed to go to the hospital. I walked over to the chair where he now spent most of his time.

He was pale and coughing up pink foamy sputum.

"I'm taking you to the hospital," I whispered and he reached out for me. He was so weak that I had to help him out of the chair and into the car.

Under most conditions, this scene would have been disturbing to me but now I was finally at peace; I finally had something that I could actually do.

As we arrived at the familiar emergency room door, I knew Rob could not make it inside by himself. I went in to get a wheelchair and told the lady at the registration desk I was bringing him in.

She instructed me to take him over to sign in, but as we crossed over the threshold and she got a glimpse of his condition, I saw the panic on her face.

People came rushing from all different directions. A stretcher, an orderly, and an MD appeared at the same time.

"We'll get him settled in," he said. "Why don't you do the paperwork and we will find him a room."

Chapter 2
Finding the Way

B eing the family member of a hospitalized patient is a stressful situation. No, let me say it in another way; it is hell.

You can hardly stand to see your loved one in that hospital bed. It brings every raw emotional feeling to the surface. Your skin is more sensitive; your heartbeat is faster, and you live in that constant state of panic. Your life is turned upside down, and the ups and downs are exhausting.

Any control you had in your life is now gone. You try to juggle your job, the kids, and everything else from the bedside, but eventually you have to leave. Then you worry even more when you aren't there.

What were they doing to him? Are they doing it correctly? Is someone checking on him? What if something happens and I am not there? Do they know he likes two pillows at night? Is he scared? Does he sense my fear?

Being at the mercy of the healthcare staff, you learn to balance your fears and concerns with smiles and silence.

The person with whom you shared your life is now in the hands of some stranger. You try to figure out who you can talk to and who you can't. You need communication from someone; anyone, but you don't know who to ask.

Feeling so helpless, you watch the reactions and the non-verbal's of the healthcare staff as they come in and out of the room because they must know what is going on. If they seem concerned, then you worry but you don't know what to worry about. If they seem okay, then you relax because things must be alright; but you aren't sure.

Do they just not know? Or care? Your mind races but you have to monitor your thoughts and actions, or you will lose any sense of reasoning and act like a fool. But sometimes you just act like a fool anyway. You are not your normal self and you wonder who this person is that came in and took over your mind.

Being assertive without making anyone pissed off is a tricky situation. And being tricky is too difficult to maneuver when your stomach is firmly planted in your throat.

By the time I found Rob's room, he was settled in and had an entourage of staff hovering over him. IV's, oxygen, and a multitude of medications were being administered.

"His weight is up so we are giving him some medications to pull the fluid off," the nurse said without looking up.

"Okay," I answered calmly as I remained back and out of the way.

I had a million questions: How much weight? What medications? Where is the doctor?

"Where the hell were all you people yesterday when I needed your help," I wanted to shout, but instead, I sat in the stained straight-backed chair over in the corner and just watched.

He looked pale and swollen, "Like the Pillsbury doughboy," I thought as I smiled.

I remembered when Rob and I would cuddle on the couch while we watched TV. When that commercial came on, he would tickle me in the stomach just like the hand on the screen.

I am so ticklish that I would scream and laugh, trying to get him to stop. We would end up on the floor rolling around like two kids until I yelled "uncle!"

The picture in my mind made me laugh inside, and I had to hold myself back in the chair to keep from climbing up in the bed with him. I wanted him to tickle me now.

My eyes began to tear up, but I forced myself to stop. I couldn't say "uncle" now. I had to hold it together for both of us. He had been the strong one but now it was my turn.

One by one, the mass of people left the room. He had been stuck, probed, measured, and medicated until there was not much left to do. His weight was up 26 pounds.

We both knew his condition had worsened but we had no idea it was this severe. Because of all the drugs given to remove the fluid, he would not get much sleep. They prepared him for the many trips to the bathroom but explained how this would take the load off his heart.

When the last nurse left the room and we were finally alone, I went over and sat on the edge of the bed. He looked so tired.

"I'm sorry," he said as he took my hand.

"Sorry?" I asked.

"Yes, sorry to put you through all this. You've had so much pain in your life already, you don't need anymore."

His words hit me like a wrecking ball swinging from a high crane and into a dilapidated old building that was hanging on by a thread—one swing and it is completely gone.

All the energy in the universe could not hold me together at this point.

I laid across his chest and sobbed those uncontrollable choking sobs that come from so deep within your soul, you fear you will never be able to stop. He patted my head and rubbed my hair until I finally settled down.

I was an "all or nothing" kind of gal. As the oldest child in an alcoholic home, I was to become a strong yet fearful, black or white, 100% or 0% adult. I would go and go and go and go… and then crash so fast, I could break the sound barrier on the way down. No middle ground for me.

I actually had a quote on my mirror at home that read, "Strive to be average." Rob knew that about me so he just waited patiently until the sobs slowly disappeared.

As I raised my head, he smiled at my red spotty face and the liquid dangling from my nose. I was a sight; I knew it. I looked at him and said, "I want to be the Pillsbury Doughboy."

He took his finger and gently poked me in the side and we both laughed. No more words needed. We would be okay. It was like playing that mental video of the building crashing down in reverse.

"Go home and take care of our boys," he said, as he headed toward the bathroom.

As I entered the room the following morning, the doctor arrived at the same time. He settled back into a chair, and I thought that was odd. Most of the time, physicians are in and out so quickly that there isn't enough time to even ask questions.

He started to talk to us about Rob's condition and how things may happen sooner rather than later. Although his weight was coming down, his condition had deteriorated and he wasn't sure how many more occurrences of heart failure Rob's body could take.

He said he had spent many hours on the phone looking for a hospital that performed heart transplants and also took insurance as payment.

This was a time when many insurance companies considered this process experimental and would not pay for the surgery. One had agreed to work him up but wanted $50,000 payment up front. Of course, this was impossible for us, and he knew that.

He then talked about a hospital about 90 minutes away. They had just begun their heart transplant program and were willing to consider Rob as a possible candidate.

It was a complicated process because you had to meet strict criteria before being considered. A psychological evaluation, a dental exam, and all sorts of tests and scans had to be completed.

This was to ensure there was no source of infection to affect the transplanted heart and that there was a personality in place that was able to handle the stress of the situation.

If you pass all of these preliminary tests, you are then placed on a waiting list. Unfortunately, some people die before a match can be found. A torturous process for such modern times.

We both sat in silence. The information was so overwhelming, even I was at a loss for words. Thoughts flew through my mind like a movie on fast forward.

How is it possible that my 34 year old sweet and gentle husband needed his heart removed from his chest and replaced with a different one in order to live? It was too much to digest.

As thoughts swirled in my head, he continued. "When this happens, I want to prepare you for all the attention this will bring. The press will contact you, follow you, and want to interview you. Think about how you want to handle this in advance. The decision is yours, but it will be better if you figure that out beforehand."

The mind is a wonderful thing. When it is so full of information that is too much to absorb and disseminate all at once, it goes into what I call "list mode."

We began making lists. Call the family. Make arrangements for the kids. Talk to my boss. Oh yeah, talk to Rob's manager. Catch up on the bills.

We spoke like we were planning a grocery store trip. Neither one of us was ready to even imagine what was ahead of us so we functioned like robots with our sanity lists grasped firmly in hand.

I left the hospital in a daze. When a loved one is ill, it affects everyone in the family. It resembles rippled water on a pond. When the stone hits the water, the disturbance moves across the entire surface, and the water underneath is in turmoil. This pretty much described our family over the next 36 hours.

I made the first phone call and the ripple effect began. The phone rang all night long and the parade of people in and out of the house was overwhelming. It wasn't like I didn't appreciate all the care and concern; I did. But my head was still in a fog and I needed time to sort it all out.

I repeated the story so many times, I wanted to just record it, put it on my voice mail, and go to bed. I wanted to wake up and tell Rob what a terrible nightmare I had that night, and then get up and go on with our lives. But this was real, and if this was going to happen any time soon, I had to make arrangements for Jeff and Adam.

After the commotion settled down, I sat down with the boys. I explained in simple terms what might happen.

It's funny how different personalities react. Adam cried and clung to my leg while Jeff was stoic and showed little outward reaction. We all ate dinner in silence.

I was off work the next day, so I got up early to get the boys off to school. I wanted their lives to be as normal as possible for as long as I could, so we kept our daily routine.

After carpooling and doing some laundry, I went to the hospital. As I entered his room and found it empty, my heart sank. I couldn't take much more.

I ran to the nurse's station. The nurses were busy so I stood at the desk and waited until one was free. I tried staring, clearing my throat, and finally saying, "Excuse me." It seemed like minutes but I am sure it was just a few seconds, and finally one looked up.

"Can I help you?" she said as she continued to work.

"Help me?" I thought. "Where the hell is Rob?" I screamed inside my head. Instead, I smiled and asked, "Can you tell me where my husband might be?"

Of course, the day shift staff had no idea who I was so we had to go through the questions and answers for them to figure out just who they were looking for and where he was.

After shuffling through papers and looking in the computer, it was determined that "room 324" had been moved to ICU early in the morning. No one could explain why I wasn't called; he was moved during the night shift and those staff members were already gone.

As I dashed up the stairs, I didn't know whether to laugh or to cry. Did these people not know that this man needed his heart replaced? That our entire lives were upside down; that I had entrusted his care to them and no one even knew where he was.

What was it going to take to get their attention? Did they even care? Have they ever had a loved one hospitalized? Were they immune to all of this? It seemed he was just a room number to them.

I pushed the entry button to the ICU and got no response. As I wondered why I even had to ask permission to see my own husband, the door clicked and I entered the intensive care unit.

I was directed to the room and as I turned the corner, guilt overcame me like a blanket of snow. Rob was in bed surrounded by four nurses, five IV's hanging with tubing draped across his chest and into his neck. How could I even think about what was happening to me when he was in this condition?

When he saw my face, he smiled and said, "I think it's a go, Hun."

"What's a go and why in the hell did I not know you were in the ICU again?" I was losing all control and I knew it.

I guess my frustration was obvious because one of the nurses immediately acknowledged me. She had a warm smile and took my hand.

"You must be Mrs. Schofield," she said. "I am Sue."

She brought a chair over to the bedside and offered it to me.

"We still have a few things to do here, but please have a seat so we can talk and work at the same time."

I immediately began to relax a little bit. She was pleasant and kind and she had a name. I finally felt like he was in good hands.

As they worked with Rob, she continued to talk.

The doctor was in early this morning with some good news. The hospital has agreed to accept your husband as a possible candidate and will begin the work up for a transplant.

He will be going tomorrow but, before that can occur, he needs some medications to keep his heart functioning well enough to tolerate the trip. He needed to be in ICU so we could monitor him more closely while on these medications.

I am sorry you were not notified; that was our mistake. We will be finished here soon and then you can have some privacy.

I melted into the chair. Letting the family know what is going on is the best customer service a hospital can provide.

Knowing we didn't have much time to prepare, my visit was brief.

Rob was being transported by helicopter the following morning, but I was unable to go with him. The area inside was small and the stretcher and transport personnel would occupy most of it.

I spent the day on the phone, making arrangements, and, in the end, it was decided that my sister, my mother-in-law, and I would travel together by car.

Adam was going to a neighbor's house and Jeff was being taken care of by a family associated with his school. I juggled my schedule to get a few days off in a row and I contacted Rob's boss. By the end of the day, everything seemed to be in place.

I took the boys to the hospital to see Rob that night and the four of us were able to spend some time together as a family. Normally children were not permitted in the ICU but they made an exception for us.

By now, the news had spread throughout the hospital that a helicopter was coming for the regions first potential heart transplant. You could hear the buzz among the staff, whispering and smiling as we walked by. Our life was now on display.

Chapter 3
Heart and Soul

*W*e got on the road about 10 a.m. the next morning. Even though it was December, it was a brisk sunny day. The conversation was light, but the concern was heavy.

Rob had been lifted from the roof of the hospital about 9 a.m. He was scheduled for a series of tests so we were told to take our time getting to the hospital.

A friend of Rob's family lived in the same city and invited the three of us to stay at her home. My plan was to spend a couple of days there during the routine testing and then go back home, so this arrangement was perfect. I was beginning to learn that making things simple is what helps families of patients.

We found Rob shortly after entering the hospital. He had completed a few tests and was preparing to go to the cath lab. He looked good and was excited to tell us about the helicopter ride.

We met many of the staff members who were assigned to care for Rob during this admission. They were warm and friendly and kept us informed. The coordinator of the heart transplant program was a nurse named Judy.

"Judy with a Y," she said smiling, referring to mine being spelled with an I.

She gave us an itinerary of what they would be doing over the next two days and a tour that helped us find our way around the hospital.

We visited with Rob between his tests, and he said he felt safe and secure here. All those medications had increased the functioning of his heart so he was alert and talkative.

After some small talk and laughter, we said our goodbyes and headed off to settle in for the night.

As we gathered around the dinner table that evening, I relaxed for the first time in months. Karen's home was cozy and comfortable, and we all felt at ease in her company. We had a glass or two of wine while sharing childhood stories and talked about the good old days.

Karen and Rob's families were long time neighbors. The kids all grew up together and remained friends as adults. She had recently married and moved away, but the minute she heard about Rob, she insisted we spend the night with her. I was glad she did.

The next morning, after going to church and breakfast, we headed to the hospital. We were all relaxed and in a pleasant but guarded mood. Things were looking good but the test results would determine the next step.

As we entered the hospital, Judy and a few others met us at the door.

"Rob has taken a turn for the worse," she began. They had waited in the lobby so they wouldn't miss us, but we were now briskly walking and talking simultaneously.

"He went into cardiac arrest this morning. We resuscitated him but he is on a ventilator and unresponsive."

She stopped and faced me, taking my hands into hers. Her face was tense and her palms were moist.

"His only chance is a new heart, but I have to tell you, he has to have that heart transplant within 24 hours or he will not make it."

As she put her arm around me, we continued to the elevator. She basically held me up as we walked, and as we entered a private conference room, my legs buckled beneath me.

Rob's mom and my sister began to cry, as I whispered, "Is that possible?"

"We have never found a heart in 24 hours" she responded hesitantly, but then adding quickly, "We have placed him at the top of the national list. His blood type is B positive, so if a heart matching that becomes available anywhere in the country, it will be his."

I am not sure I can adequately describe the feeling that follows that type of news. An internal shaking begins deep inside like an earthquake preparing to explode through the surface of the earth. The mouth becomes parched, the heart pounds, and thoughts swirl so fast in your head, you become breathless and nauseated. The tears are the last to surface.

I tried to hold it together but when I looked over at the face of his mother, I lost all control. The pain was so deep, my soul ached with sorrow.

The staff supported us with tissues and hugs until we were able to comprehend the reality of all this. "Can I see him?" I murmured between those gasps of breaths you take after a sobbing cry.

"Of course," Judy said as she led me to the room.

Rob was in ICU. The room was dim, but I could see his face from the doorway. There was a tube in his mouth that was connected to the ventilator and several IV drips. His chest rose with every push of artificial air from the machine and fell as the air escaped from his mouth.

I took his hand in mine as I rubbed his forehead.

"Please wake up Rob. I can't do this on my own," I begged. Then the guilt crept into every cell of my being. How could I be thinking about me again when he was on the brink of death? How could I have had fun last night, even drinking wine and laughing while Rob needed me here? I should have never left; should've, could've, would've. Guilt is a common denominator in families of critically ill patients. We wear a veil of Guilt.

As my sister and mother-in-law went to the bedside, I began making the calls back home. The rest of the family had to be notified, and I needed to talk to my children.

The caravan of relatives began as the word spread, and Rob had a sister living outside the U.S. who was trying to get home as well. I was now doing okay because I was in "list phase," but when I heard my son's voice on the phone, the reality of the situation became apparent again.

Thoughts circulated around like a wind tunnel, and words and half sentences stumbled out in between tears. Being that person who needs control, I wanted to lasso in this whole situation and jerk it back into place, but instead, I just sat. It was out of my hands and in the hands of the medical staff. Did they know how much we depend on their expertise and hope for an ounce of human kindness?

The family all eventually gathered in a comfortable waiting room. As each one arrived, someone would take on the task of updating them and then taking them to see Rob. The reaction was always the same; quietly wiping tears as they came back to our gathering place.

There is strength in numbers during these situations and we were grateful for the thoughtful amenities that our new friends provided; coffee, a phone, and frequent visits to see how we were doing.

Judy was our lifeline connection. If there was any change at all, she immediately came to update us; even if there was no new information, she would just sit and talk.

The next time Judy entered the room, I knew something had changed. Her demeanor and her facial expression were different. I held my breath as she announced there was a possible donor. Snippets of her next sentences were all I heard; a possible donor, a vehicle accident, a young man from Minnesota, type B.

After a wave of gratitude and a silent word of thanks, I thought of that other family. They were in the same situation as us but their outcome was not good. I whispered a quiet prayer for them and then tried to come back to the present.

The process included tissue sampling and donor surgery, so we would not have an answer for a few hours, but the outlook was good. The atmosphere immediately changed. There were conversations and even a laugh or two heard across the room. Everyone was making phone calls to update those at home. Hope is a good thing.

The emotional rollercoaster over the next few hours was unbearable. A blizzard in Minnesota delayed the plane, and when the samples arrived, some were mistakenly frozen and could not be used. The family donated many organs so the body was in surgery for a few hours, and the heart was the last thing to be removed.

In the meantime, Rob's condition was deteriorating and time was not on our side. With each changing situation, the staff would bring us the news. Keeping us informed was a priority, and we were grateful for it.

The last visit brought good news and bad news. The heart was finally on its way but Rob was now so critical, something needed to be done immediately.

After he had coded again, the decision was made to take him to surgery. They would open his chest, place him on the bypass machine, and hopefully keep him alive until the heart arrived. This was not a typical procedure, but Rob was going to die without it, so it was a last chance decision.

I was taken to a small room with Judy and a few other staff members. They explained that since Rob was unable to speak for himself, I had to sign the consent forms for his surgery.

As I looked at the large stack of papers they had before them, fear overcame me. Death, stroke, moon face; the list was just beginning. The consent forms covered the heart transplant and all the possible side effects of the medications he would be on for the rest of his life. That is, if he lived.

The reading continued for 10 minutes, but it seemed like a lifetime.

Being an LPN, I knew in my head that they had to present any possible problem that may occur, but as a wife, my heart was so distressed. Could I make such an important decision? What if he had brain damage? What if…what if…

Suddenly I said, "I want to talk to my mom." When we are under stress, we revert back to our childish ways. That is why many family members lose all good sense and act out in ways that they normally would not when their loved one is sick.

I called my mom; she was at home and unable to make the trip down. We talked and cried, and in the end, I signed all the papers. As I headed back to my family, I was still questioning whether I had done the right thing. Exhaustion takes over any sense of decision making.

The mood in the room was somber. A few had gone to the chapel; others were stretched across the chairs. Rob was in the OR; the heart was in transit. No one even knew if it was a good match but it didn't matter; we were in checkmate now.

Earlier, the hospital asked if I was interested in speaking to a reporter from the local newspaper. He wanted to follow a heart transplant case from beginning to end, and, after meeting him and discussing with my family, I agreed. We decided any information shared with others could only help the heart transplant program.

He was a wonderful man who sat and waited with us and got to know my family on a personal level. As he and his photographer left to prepare for the OR, Judy and her staff passed out hugs and promised frequent updates. All that was left for us to do now was to wait and pray.

Over the next few hours, the nurses and the rest of the staff made frequent visits to keep us informed. It was probably the one thing that kept us from completely falling apart. They considered our needs an important part of the process and understood the role family played in the care of the patient.

On the final visit, the news was good and bad yet again. Rob had coded another time before the surgery began, but the heart arrived and was successfully placed in his chest. It was not known if Rob went without oxygen long enough to cause brain damage, but the new heart was beating.

The reporter told me later that the old heart was found to be so enlarged when it was removed, it would not fit in the surgical basin. He also said as they wheeled Rob from the surgical suite, the anesthesiologist yelled, "Robert!! Robert Schofield! Open your eyes!!" He wanted to see if Rob was conscious.

He said Rob had opened his eyes on his command so that was a good sign. We absorbed the good news and rejected the bad; our emotional bucket was just too full.

The surgeon took all of us into a private room. He explained the entire surgery in layman's terms and said Rob was critical but presently stable.

My sister-in-law hugged him as the photographer snapped their picture, and, as we looked back at it later, they both were smiling and crying at the same time. The entire staff was as emotional as us. It had been a long day for everyone and even a little success was celebrated together.

As we left that room, I suddenly stopped and listened.....beep, beep, beep. It was the sound of the heart monitor on Rob beeping at a strong steady pace. The same familiar monitor sound I had heard so many times before in the ICU.

I looked down the hall and Rob was being wheeled into the cardiac ICU. As I walked toward the sound, his eyes turned slowly toward me and he gave me a slight thumb's up. My husband had a new heart and he recognized me by sight. Nothing else mattered as I fell into my sister's arms and sobbed tears of joy that came from the deepest part of my being.

Chapter 4

Coming Home

R ob's recovery was dramatic. Although he remained in the ICU for a couple of weeks, he was very stable. He began receiving all the anti-rejection medications so he was vulnerable to infections. I was allowed to visit him for 30 minutes four times a day, so I spent most of my time in the waiting room.

My sister went home to get me some clothes, and I had to figure out how to manage all of this. Job, kids, financial concerns, the press; I tried to handle it all.

In the end, I would go home and work three twelve-hour shifts in a row. The boys would come home and life would be somewhat normal for them during those three days; but just when they were settling in, they were uprooted again. The neighbors would take them back to their respective homes while I headed back to the hospital for the other four days of the week. Turmoil was our middle name.

There seemed to be no ill effects from the surgery. Rob was doing well, and 27 days after the heart transplant, he came home.

All the staff at the hospital were excellent. They kept us informed and considered the entire family in all decisions. The discharge teaching was geared toward all of our needs, and they provided it a little at a time so we could absorb and understand it.

The day we left, the entire medical staff came to tell us goodbye. Rob was a walking miracle but they always made it a point to compliment me on my support and strength as well. They were truly our guardian angels.

As Rob and I headed north on the expressway, I looked over at him napping in the passenger seat.

"What the hell just happened here?" I thought. "My husband has another person's heart in his chest. His medications would be over $600.00 a month and I have two kids to put through school. Will he ever be able to work again? Would we lose our little house? What if I get sick?"

I had to purposefully stop this thought process. It did no good to worry-it would not change the outcome.

He glanced over at me and smiled, and I saw the assurance in his eyes that he was okay because I was—or so it seemed. I knew then that I had to be the rock—the pillar that supported us all.

I used to look to him for my strength but now our roles were reversed. Everyone was looking toward me, and I couldn't let them down.

We had experienced such marvelous medical care despite my mini breakdowns and snappy attitude at times. They understood my fear and the impact of Rob's illness on our lives. I just assumed all medical personnel performed in the same manner and with the same professionalism as our new friends, and I valued their warm and caring ways. We owed them our lives. Gratitude replaced guilt.

Over the next few weeks, there were plenty of ups and downs. Trying to find the right dose of medications was a complicated process for any patient, and Rob was no exception.

One night as the boys and I were watching TV, we heard a thud. We found Rob unconscious and on the floor. He was flown back down to the hospital for testing, so I was on the road again. This time, I went down and back in the same day because I had to work and be there for Jeff and Adam.

On one of my visits, I entered his room during meal time. When he saw me, he smiled and told me that he was allowed to order anything on the menu.

"This steak is delicious," he said as he raised the fork to his mouth "You want a bite?"

My first reaction was to take that plate of food and dump it on the floor.

"How dare he," I thought. I was totally exhausted from working full time, keeping up our family and the house, and getting down every other day to see him, and here he was, sitting up in bed eating steak without a care in the world.

Although I didn't share my feelings with him, I cut that visit short. But on the way home, my friend Guilt came back to visit me again.

"How can you even begin to feel this way after all he has been through?" I heard as I looked over at the passenger seat as if the emotional voice was a real person. Before I could justify a response, Guilt answered for me, "you should be ashamed of yourself."

I cried all the way home, and I am sure the cars passing me wondered what would make someone go into the "ugly cry" while driving down I-71. It was de je vu all over again.

When I was at the hospital, I wanted to be home with my sons; when I was home, I wanted to be with Rob. But no matter where I was, Guilt was always by my side.

Another time, Rob started vomiting blood and had to be rushed back to the hospital. This time it was a side effect of all the steroids he had to take, and the diagnosis was a bleeding ulcer. He remained hospitalized for a few days until they could begin to heal the ulcer and give him blood to replenish what he had lost.

During this hospitalization, Rob and I had a long talk. He began by talking about his insurance papers and his files at home. When I tried to stop him, he explained that he saw what this was doing to me.

"You have all the worry and work and all I have to do is lay here and get better."

Just knowing he understood that made all the difference in the world. When patients and their loved ones keep the communication open, the stress level is lowered.

We talked for hours that evening about everything from what flowers to plant in the yard next spring to his living will requests. We shared great quality time that day, and Guilt went on a well-needed vacation for a while.

Even with all these setbacks, Rob was recuperating very well. Every six weeks, he had to make a trip to the hospital for a biopsy of his heart. A device would be placed in his neck and threaded down to his heart, and small snip-its of his heart muscle would be examined for rejection. Based on those results, the medications would then be adjusted.

He and I would make a day of it. After the procedure, we would go to lunch and then visit with the staff and other patients waiting for a heart. Rob looked so healthy, and it was amazing to watch the faces of those patients light up when he told his story to them.

"If I can do it, so can you," he would say with that cute smile of his, and I could tell they really did believe him.

The last thing we would do is go to his doctor's visit. I was always included in the conversation because they believed that in order to practice holistic medicine, you treat the family as well. I was always asked if I had any questions, and all conversations were directed to both of us.

I recently had read about a survey that examined how much information patients and their families retained after a physician would speak with them. What they discovered was that patients and families usually had a question or a concern that worried them. Until the doctor got to that topic in the conversation, they retained little of what was said beforehand. The answer, it seemed, was simple; just ask the questions first.

When the physician would begin the conversation by addressing their concerns first and then proceeding with the other information, they were able to relax and absorb all that was explained.

Our visits were just like this. At the time, I took it for granted and didn't realize just how unusual it really was.

The press followed Rob wherever he went, and going back to work was no exception. They were outside the house when he arrived home from the transplant; they had a picture of him working in his garden; and they went to his workplace the day he returned there. Rob was warm and friendly to them and tried to answer all their questions.

During one interview, someone asked him if he still loved his wife. Puzzled, he asked why he would ask such a question. The reporter went on to say since love was associated with the heart and he now had some-one else's, did he still love the same people he did before the transplant. We laughed all the way home.

Rob had his surgery in December, and he was back to work by March. He was so happy to feel productive again, and the staff greeted him with a warm welcome. I was pretty nervous about it all but when I saw the positive effect it had on him, I calmed down. I have to admit, though, it was hard to relax.

I worked from 8 a.m. until 8 p.m., and Rob worked eight hour days. He and the kids would have dinner together on my work days and save me food for later.

A few times I would arrive home in the evening to a quiet house.

"Rob," I would say as I walked through the house. With each empty room I entered, my heart raced, my breathing became shallow while my voice cracked, and, in the back of my mind, I was expecting to find him passed out on the floor.

Finally he would come walking through the door telling me what a good time he and Adam had fishing or something like that, and then my body would just deflate like a balloon with a hole in it. The ups and downs were dramatic.

Eventually things fell back into that controlled chaotic routine. Jeff graduated from high school and was looking at colleges; Adam completed kindergarten and was preparing for the first grade. Rob and I both continued to work and live day to day as if everything was normal…but normal it wasn't.

The anti-rejection medications that he had to take were expensive and had significant side effects. Rob was susceptible to infections and had major mood swings plus an insatiable appetite. We continued our 90 mile trek every six weeks and were always nervous until the results were in.

One day Rob announced at the dinner table "I think we should move."

I laughed, thinking this was one of his altered mood thoughts and "this too shall pass," but it did not. He argued that the neighborhood was changing and he didn't want to raise Adam in this environment.

I talked to Judy and the doctors on our next visit, and they saw no reason not to go for it.

"Life expectancy is at least five years and by then, there will be more research extending it even more."

Reluctantly I went house shopping with him and we found a cute little "fixer upper" we both liked and could afford. We made an offer and in July, moved into our home. That night we forgot about all the boxes that needed unpacking. Instead, we sat out on the dilapidated deck and toasted to our future.

A few weeks later, on a warm August day, the four of us packed up and moved Jeff off to college. Going to Vanderbilt in Nashville, he was really excited but a little nervous. After we got him settled in and said our tearful good byes, we headed back home as a threesome.

The next week Adam entered the first grade and Rob and I talked about our "empty nest" and what we might want to plan for us in the future. We missed our kids but looked forward to some time together as a couple.

We had taken a few vacations to Myrtle Beach in the past, but now we had a lofty goal—we wanted to go to Hawaii. It would be financially impossible right now, but it was fun talking about it. And it was stress relief from all the changes in our lives.

The following Tuesday, Rob called me at work. I was so busy and aggravated when I answered the phone. He told me a friend had invited him to the race track this particular night and would it be alright if he left Adam at a neighbor's house. I guess I was less than excited about his plans, because I found out later that he did not go.

"Do whatever you want Rob, I am busy," was my response as I hung up quickly. Everyone at one time or another has those kinds of conversations with the people they love, but what I didn't know was that this time it would be my last one with Rob.

Chapter 5
The Final Call

"You need to come home. Your husband is sick." The voice was my neighbor's and for a moment, I thought it was a joke. The office was busy and when I answered the phone, I didn't recognize the person on the other end.

"What?" I gasped.

"You need to come home," she said with panic in her voice.

I grabbed my purse and yelled to my peers as I ran out the door, "It's Rob." My legs were trembling and I was unable to concentrate as I grasped the wheel with white knuckles and yelled out loud to no one in the car.

"What am I going to do? Please let him be okay. Did he go to the race track? Is Adam with him? I'm sorry I was rude on the phone Rob. Please talk to me. Please be able to talk to me. Oh my God, I am so sorry I was rude on the phone!"

I don't remember the rest of the drive but suddenly I realized I was home. As I pulled up in front of the house, an ambulance was in the driveway and a few curious neighbors had gathered on the walk.

I ran up the side yard and found the paramedics performing CPR on Rob as they were carrying the stretcher down toward me. I froze in place as they passed by me and indicated that I should follow them. They placed him in the back and led me to the front seat with the driver. I was functioning mechanically, not uttering a word. The silence was deafening and it felt like we were moving in slow motion.

The driver finally looked over and said, "They are doing everything they can for him." I almost laughed. She had no idea. My mind was swimming with thoughts and questions and memories. I wasn't even sure what to pray for.

When I saw him on the stretcher, I knew it was bad. If they resuscitated him and he would have to be on life support, he would never forgive me.

"I'll come back and haunt you," he said smiling one day when we were talking about this very subject.

But I just couldn't let him go... not yet... I can't... I just can't. Help me God. Please help.

As the siren screeched and we sped toward the hospital, thoughts began flashing through my head like a movie trailer. One question after another: What do I pray for? Where is my son? Can I make my first house payment? Who will call Jeff? Is Rob in pain? Why was I so abrupt on the phone? Was he mad at me? Why didn't he go to the race track with his friend? How long is it going to take to get to the hospital?

I could hear the thumps of the CPR still being performed on him in the back of the ambulance and my heart ached to an internal depth I had never known. I had so many things I needed to tell him: his mom had called and invited us to dinner; the car insurance company wants to update our policy; Jeff is coming home for Thanksgiving; Adam rode the school bus by himself for the first time.

I then moved straight to the "bargaining" phase of grief; "I promise God, if you give Rob back to me, I will never talk to anyone on the phone like that again. I promise... and I'll give more money to the church, and I'll….the list making went on until we arrived at the ER entrance.

Rob was whisked off through the back door and I was directed to the registration desk. My entire body was shaking and my mouth was parched.

I looked around and the waiting room was over-flowing with people. I was in the midst of a large crowd but so very alone. I wanted my family, my sister, my mom. The clerk asked me to sign in and give her some information.

"Can I use your phone?" I asked. "I need to call my family." Cell phones were not allowed inside the hospital at that time and I needed to connect with my family.

"I will get you a phone when we are finished ma'am." She was nice and professional in her encounter with me, but I knew she did not know the magnitude of my pain and potential loss. She couldn't have known or she would have understood my urgency, right?

Being a health care worker, I knew the registration routine and the importance of insurance information and signatures. We did it every day. It wasn't that I didn't want to complete it; I just wanted to make one call before we started.

I asked again with a cracked voice, "Can I please call my sister?"

"Yes ma'am, as soon as I can get your information."

I know that the emergency room registers a large number of people, and I am sure they hear every story that could be imagined, but when it is your husband and your situation, you want the encounter to be personal.

As I was searching for my insurance card, a nurse appeared from the back and asked the clerk "Is anyone here with the code?"

"The code?" I panicked. Is she talking about Rob? I stood up and immediately said, "Do you mean Rob? His name is Rob! I am here. Is he okay? I am here with the code… I mean Rob!"

My reaction startled her, and she said she would go check on him and left me standing with all eyes focused on me and my outburst. I sat back down and completed the paperwork as she requested, and then I was finally given the desk phone to use. I would have preferred a more private place, but I was just grateful to have a phone.

I made one call to each side of the family and asked them to pass on the information. Everyone in the ER could hear me so I tried not to cry when I made the calls.

As I hung up the phone, I could feel all the eyes focused on me, whispering and trying to figure out what was going on. I stood there, not sure where to go or what to do.

There was nowhere to sit, and I was doing everything in my power not to stand in the middle of the waiting room and cry. So I paced. Up and down; back and forth. A few people would smile as I passed them, wanting to say something but not sure what.

What a relief it was when my family started trickling in! My brother-in law arrived first, followed by my sister and a few of Rob's other siblings. I grabbed on to them and cried as each one arrived and repeated what little information I had to share.

Soon we had quite a crowd standing in the waiting room. The ER was very busy, so no one was available to tell us what to do. Finally, a nursing supervisor came to see what she could do to help. This was possibly the death of my young precious husband and I did not want to experience it in the middle of a crowded waiting room.

She found us a nice room that had a phone and some bottled water and she came back a few times to check on us. As I sat there, I reflected on the last week—wondering if I had missed some sign; some signal that something wasn't right.

The weekend before, Rob had connected with his good friend from the past, and they had gone fishing. He came back with a string full of fish that he swung in my face to aggravate me. I reacted more than I normally would just because I knew that is what he wanted me to do. He laughed out loud as he headed off for the cleaning process.

The next Saturday we attended his cousin's wedding. He got to spend time with all of his relatives that he had not seen in a while, and we had the best time. We laughed until our stomachs hurt and we danced our feet off. On the way home, he said he couldn't remember when he had so much fun.

That Sunday, we had my best friend and her fiancé over for dinner. Rob grilled some wonderful tuna, and we ate until we were stuffed. It was a great time and we were so happy that the guys really got along so well.

Monday he had taken my car and had four tires put on it. "They looked worn so I just replaced them all," he said when he returned. Nothing out of the ordinary.

That night as we prepared for bed, he stopped and turned to look at me.

"I love you," he said softly.

"I love you too," I replied matter of factly. He took me by the shoulders and looked me straight in the eyes.

"No, I mean I REALLY love you." He almost sounded desperate for me to understand.

"Okay," I said and gave him a hug. "I really love you too." Did he know? Did he have some kind of premonition?

It all started to make sense. He recently took the opportunity to see longtime family and friends, and it was like he got the rest of us settled in before he could go.

We got Jeff off to Vanderbilt, Adam into the first grade, moved to a nicer neighborhood—oh my God, I wonder if he knew! Why didn't he talk to me about it?

"I'll have to ask him when I finally get to see him," I thought to myself as I denied the inevitable.

It seemed like forever since we had arrived, but finally the door opened. A man came into the conference room wearing blue scrub pants, a white tee shirt, and suspenders. He did not identify himself, but instead said, "Mrs. Schofield?"

I stood in the middle of the room, not sure what to expect. I stared at his face. I didn't know who he was, but whoever he was, I wanted to hear from him that Rob was doing well and I could go see him. I waited for the words to come from his mouth.

Instead, I heard a flat monotone voice say, "Your husband is dead. He was dead before he ever hit the door, but the official time of death will be 8:15 p.m."

The silence was horrible. I wanted to scream but nothing would come out. It was like being in that dream state when you try to shout but can't and you wake up in a cold sweat.

We stood like two soldiers at attention until I finally whispered, "Can I see him?"

"Yes," he said. "The nurse will come and get you in a few minutes after they clean him up." He turned and walked out the door.

Chapter 6
Sticks and Stones

I have a theory I call the "Invisible Suitcase" theory. I believe we all walk around with our "invisible baggage" strapped on our back. Finances, relationships, work, children, and a boat load of other things that we worry about on a daily basis are in this bag, and we take it with us wherever we go.

How many times have you had an argument with your spouse and then gone to work in a bad mood? The way you interacted with others that day was affected by the baggage you took out the door that morning. No one really knows what you have packed up that day or if you are traveling light or heavy at any given time.

Some people have more baggage than a Delta kiosk, and what they carry affects every aspect of their life. How we relate to each other is influenced by the load we carry to each interaction. We are not just our physical appearance but we are also what we carry around in our invisible bag.

I was no exception. My suitcase was bulging at the seams and, as I stood in the middle of that room, the contents began to overflow and I was frozen in time. I had no idea what to do next.

Finally, I turned and faced my family. Rob's mother was crying. I went to her and we hugged each other gently.

"A mother should not have to bury a child," she whispered. I couldn't even imagine how that must feel as I thought of Jeff and Adam.

"Dead," I thought and said aloud. What a cold word that person used to describe such a vibrant young man. I could not comprehend the meaning. We had plans, a future. Now our life together was no more.

We had a 30-year mortgage, college tuition, credit cards, and I was making $8.00 an hour. Could we…I mean, could I… even make the first house payment? Would we lose our house? Could Jeff continue to go to school in Nashville?

How am I going to tell this news to Jeff over the phone? I don't even know where Adam is. He is such a cute little guy who loves his dad so much. What do I do now? Tonight? Tomorrow? My baggage overflowed.

It seemed a strange time to worry about money but when we are in stressful circumstances, everything in our invisible suitcase becomes too heavy to carry. Being a 40-year old widow with two children and a small income was not in my packing plans.

A few minutes later, a nurse entered the room. "Are you ready to come back with me?" she asked in a low voice. A few of us walked to the trauma room where Rob had been taken, and as we entered the room, I saw my sweet precious Rob lying on a stretcher with a crisp white sheet pulled up to his chin.

I pulled a chair up and sat by his side and held his hand. It was still warm. His wedding ring was still on his finger and I nervously twisted it back and forth. One by one, family members came in and out, saying their last goodbyes. There were tears and hugs and offers of sympathy and assistance. Although I appreciated it, I didn't want help. I wanted my husband.

Our parish priest came, and we gathered around Rob and said some prayers. I couldn't pray, but I stood and bowed my head in respect.

Suddenly I felt like I was going to be sick and I looked for the closest restroom. As I turned the corner, I heard a conversation between two nurses who were discussing my situation.

"What the heck did she expect?" one said. "He had a heart transplant, for God's sake!"

"Yes," said the other one. "She was fortunate to have him for the extra time he did get. I can't believe that this is a surprise. I was here when he was flown down for that transplant and she is lucky he survived all that."

I came to a stop and listened.

"What did I expect??!!" I screamed silently. "What I expected was to have a normal life just like everyone else. What I expected was to have many years together, sharing grandchildren and going to Hawaii. How DARE they make assumptions about my life as to what I should feel and not feel! And LUCKY?! I should feel lucky? Lucky that Rob was soon to be put on a slab and placed in a refrigerator?

As I returned to the room, another staff member was in there asking how much longer we might be. The emergency room was busy and they needed the space as soon as we were ready to leave.

"But take as much time as you need," she said hesitantly.

"Time," I thought. How much time does it take to say goodbye to a life? To complete all the unfinished conversations and plans that happened in day to day life. To say all the things I meant to say but didn't. To apologize for not being there when I was too tired or just in a bad mood. To say 'I love you' one more time. To be the Pillsbury Doughboy.

I asked everyone to give me a minute alone with Rob. I looked around the room and I saw his personal belongings and clothes crumpled up in a chair over in the corner. I picked them up one by one and cradled them to my chest. It looked like junk to anyone else, but to me these things were more precious than gold.

The flannel shirt was the one his mom had given him for Christmas.

It still smelled like him. These were the jeans that he had just talked about on Monday.

"They have been washed enough now that they finally feel comfortable," he said as he slipped them on that morning. The wallet had pictures of the kids and his shoes still had mud from the backyard soccer game.

I was so upset that someone had not thought his personal belongings were important enough to fold up and place in a bag. I considered them sacred pieces of our life and I folded them up with the respect and dignity they deserved. Personal belongings not only have an owner, but a family and a memory attached to them as well.

I then sat by his side and tried to say my goodbye. I looked at his body, now becoming cold and stiff.

"Where are you, Rob? I know this is just the shell that housed your spirit but where did you go? I hope it is not too far. Please stay close and help me because I am not sure I can do this alone. I will take care of your boys to the best of my ability but I am scared. I am sorry Rob. I am so sorry I was rude on the phone. If I had only known"…..the door opened.

"Mrs. Schofield, we really do need this room." I bent down and kissed his lips.

"I love you Rob," I said softly crying. I then gathered up the belongings and left the room.

Most of the family had already left, but one of my neighbors had stayed behind to drive me home. I immediately asked about Adam and she said he was safe. Her daughter had taken him to her house when the ambulance arrived. I sunk into the seat and sobbed.

When we arrived home, I found all my family and some friends gathered there. Traditions are a funny thing. Often when others had an illness or death, I would go to their house and offer food and fellowship. I would stay a few hours and then go back to my normal routine, not thinking much about it.

However, when I was on the receiving end of that tradition, I realized the value of it. My family had stopped along the way and picked up refreshments and snacks. We all gathered in my little house and shared stories about Rob and some of the good times they had with him.

We laughed, cried, talked, drank beer, and just spent time supporting each other in this time of grief. There is strength in numbers. If I had to come home from the hospital to an empty house, I am not sure I could have made it through the night.

Instead, my family helped me to deal with this situation by spending time with me and sharing stories that helped me realize how important Rob was to them as well. I felt supported and loved.

I functioned over the next few days like this was just a bad dream and it would eventually end. When I talked about Rob, I spoke in present tense, not yet making the transition in my mind that he was gone.

I believe that the rituals we use at the end of life are more for those left behind than for those who have passed away. Although our intent is to honor their life, the ceremony actually gives us time to start the process of closure to one part of our life and begin the grieving process in order to move forward. It gives us sharing time with others before we have to face the aloneness of the loss. This is difficult enough without the added burden of a negative death memory.

During the next few weeks after Rob's death, I could not get the words and actions of the healthcare workers out of my mind. I thought of Judy and all the other staff who helped care for Rob during his heart transplant and remembered that as such a positive experience.

Both situations were extremely stressful, but what made this one so negative? Was it the situation or the interactions with the people? Was it my perception? I do know that the words that are spoken in any health care relationship are ingrained in the patient and the family's mind and they become part of that experience forever.

Although it occurred several years ago, I can still repeat every word that was said to me in both situations; remember the smells, picture the clothes they had on, and describe the look of the room. Words spoken during times of grief become part of the death memory for that family.

It bothered me so much that a few weeks later I decided to go back to that hospital and attempt to talk to those who were there the day Rob died. I needed to tell them how their words affected me not only that day, but every day forward.

The day I went to the emergency room, three of those employees were there. They were reluctant to speak to me, but when they realized I wasn't leaving until they did, they agreed to meet with me.

The physician remembered me and the experience of Rob's death immediately. I told him what it was like when he came into the room where we were gathered dressed the way he was and not even identifying himself.

He listened and nodded his head as I was speaking. He told me he knew he had not handled the situation wisely but that this was the first time he had to deal with the death of such a young man and he didn't know what to do.

"When your husband died under my care, I felt responsible. Young healthy men are not supposed to die. We are trained to save lives and when I couldn't do that, I didn't know what to do. I knew you were in that room and I dreaded the task of coming in and telling you. I wanted to get in and out as quickly as possible because I was so upset, and I was in scrubs because during the emergency, my clothes were soiled. I am so sorry I put my needs above yours. I didn't even realize that my actions would affect you so dramatically. Your coming here has helped me realize the importance of our interactions with families. I can't change what I said and did but I can make sure I don't repeat it again."

I was stunned. I had never even considered that the reason for his actions were his own personal struggles with Rob's death. People don't realize that the interactions health care workers have with patients and their families affect them personally as well.

His genuine expression of his feelings caused us both to cry as we hugged each other.

"I am sorry," he said.

"So am I," I answered. "I judged you without even knowing you."

I then found two of the nurses who had that conversation in the hallway the day Rob died. When I repeated what they had said that day, they didn't even remember speaking those words.

"We deal with so many people and situations here in the emergency room that if we don't vent to each other, we wouldn't be able to continue in this job. We were probably as upset as the doctor was about witnessing the death of such a young man.

Sometimes we say things to try to justify in our minds some of the situations we see on a day to day basis here. I guess we never even thought about the fact that you could have heard us talking or that what we said would even matter to you."

We all stood in silence for a few seconds as we contemplated the reactions of each other. They were putting themselves in my place as a wife who had just lost her husband and heard caretakers voicing their opinion on the situation, while I imagined how hard it must be to be in this situation as a nurse and stay unaffected by all of it.

We talked for a few more minutes as I thanked them for allowing me to come to their workplace and express my feelings, and they said they were grateful that I did.

I left there feeling like a big burden had been lifted off my mind and now I could begin my grieving process without this excess baggage. Communication in any healthcare situation is vital to the success of the interaction.

Healthcare workers need to know how we hang on to every verbal and non-verbal communication we have with them, and how they interact with us has a dramatic effect on the reactions of the patient and the family.

On the other hand, the patient and the family need to realize that medical personnel are doing the best they can under some stressful situations, and that before we judge them, we should try to understand their side of each situation.

As I walked to my car, the clouds began to part and the sun shone brightly through their midst. I felt the warmth of the rays wrap around me on this October day, and I smiled for the first time since Rob's death as I looked up.

"Thank you Rob. I know you are with me," I whispered, as I headed home to begin the grieving process.

Part Two:

The Nurse's View

"In the sick room, ten cents' worth of human under-standing equals ten dollars' worth of medical science."

— Martin H. Fischer

Chapter 7

Nurses' Notes

"When I open my hospital, families will not be allowed," I stated boldly to my co-worker one day at work.

The minute the words came out of my mouth, I had to laugh at myself. How soon we forget our past experiences and fall into the trappings of the current day situations.

I was now working as a registered nurse in a hospital cardiac unit, and it had been a rough day. As I stood in the middle of the nurse's station, I reflected on how I had gotten to this point.

At Rob's funeral, I remember hearing two things. The first was, "What can I do for you?" One after another, people asked me what I needed from them. I don't know if they said it just to be nice or if they really wanted to know, but my answer was always the same.

"Call me in six months." I meant it literally.

I knew that for the first few months everyone would be around to support us, but eventually people migrate back to their routine lives. It's just the normal thing to do. The hole in my heart was so huge that I wasn't sure I could make it alone, and asking people to remember me was my way of reaching out.

The second thing people said as they came to pay their respects was, "I guess Jeff will be moving back here to help you now." I glanced over at him a few times and saw the look on his face; the thought had never occurred to him until now.

Finally, I had to take him aside and reassure him I would be okay. Even though I didn't know how I was going to function in this world without Rob, I was rational enough to know it wasn't Jeff's responsibility to fill the void.

"You are not my husband; you are my son," I said. "You deserve to have your own life. You will go back to school and we will figure this all out together."

Within a few months, both had become a reality. Most of our friends and family settled back into their busy lives, and we tried to do the same. Jeff and Adam returned to school, and I went back to my job, but we were all on autopilot.

On the surface, I seemed to be managing things, but inside, I felt like a fish out of water. It is said that no major decisions should be made during the first year after the loss of a spouse because you believe you are thinking rationally, but in reality, you are not. However, I knew I had to make a decision about how I was going to support my family because my current income did not meet my bills.

I remember the exact moment when I made that decision. I was checking the Sunday want-ads when I saw a listing for a hospice nurse. Because of the experiences we had encountered during Rob's illness and death, the thought of helping someone else through that process seemed right.

I called for an interview and was told they did not hire LPNs, only registered nurses (RN).

"I guess I will have to go back to school," I said to myself as I hung up the phone. Then I sat down and cried; cried out of fear, and anger and frustration.

I looked around at the house that we were so excited about fixing up together and the task at hand seemed monumental. Now I was considering adding school to the mix.

"It's a good thing you are dead, Rob, because if you were here, I'd have to kill you for leaving me like this." Even I had to smile at my irrational expression of grief.

After overcoming several obstacles, I finally went back to school. My SAT scores were so outdated, I was required to re-take the test. Financial aid, work, class schedules, and child care were just a few considerations, but eventually it all fell into place.

Adjusting to the hectic requirements of nursing school helped to divert the emotional turmoil, but the raw feelings were always close at hand. One of the first clinical rotations I had was at the hospital where Rob had died, so that was a difficult day, but I was determined to see it through.

Adam and I would hang our report cards on the refrigerator, and then call Jeff to compare all of our grades. Even at age 40, I "gave them a run for their money," as the saying goes.

Looking back, I am not sure how it all came together, but three years later, I graduated. Although my original goal was to work in hospice care, I was drawn to cardiac nursing during school.

I was accepted into a critical care internship at a local hospital which gave me the opportunity to work with heart patients. Making a difference was important to me, and in some strange way, it kept me close to Rob. Things have a way of coming full circle, and now I was on the other side.

No class or book work could have ever prepared me for bedside nursing. It is a job like no other, and most people do not understand the complexity of it. There are many important positions and roles in healthcare, but nursing is at the heart of it all.

Nurses are with their patients 24 hours a day and are the liaison between all the players in the medical field.

They have to balance the complicated physical processes of each patient and be the advocate for their safe care. Nurses observe symptoms, interpret lab and test results, communicate with doctors, perform intricate procedures, offer emotional support, provide continuous education, and complete mounds of legally required charting.

On any given day, it is common to have their hands on every section of the human anatomy and in body fluids too numerous to mention. Most work twelve hour shifts, which usually end up being thirteen or more, and the majority of that time is spent on their feet. Back injuries and varicose veins are commonplace.

Lunch is a luxury, and there is an actual syndrome called nurse's bladder because of the length of time between bathroom breaks. Nurses organize, plan, care, decide, critically think, and balance information for each individual while trying to please patients, families, other health care professionals and administration.

No matter how many years of seniority or work experience, the bedside nurse is expected to be on-call and work weekends, holidays, and overtime. But despite all of this, most nurses absolutely love what they do and could not imagine doing anything else.

It is not a job but a calling.

"Being a nurse is not what I do; it is what I am," I once said and I was sincere in my description.

One particular day had been a challenge from the start. We began the day with a staff meeting which is stressful in itself. These meetings are a great way to keep nurses informed but they are also a burden as they delay the start of the workday.

It's the best way nurses can keep up with all the new information they need to hear, though, since it is a 24/7 profession. There are regulatory bodies that dictate nursing practice, and all nurses have to stay up to date on any new information.

In addition, nurses are required to have continuing education credits for their license renewal every other year, so educational offerings are provided on occasion. This, along with all the new technology and equipment that is used in healthcare, makes it necessary to have on going informational meetings.

As I was rustling around in my seat in the back of the room, I received a call from the desk. All four of my assigned patients for that day had something going on that needed my immediate attention.

Half grateful for the excuse to leave the meeting and half apprehensive of what I would find out on the unit, I soon discovered I was in over my head.

One patient was confused and climbing out of bed, the second one was having some irregular heartbeats and feeling nauseous, the third had chest pain he labeled a number 7 out of 10 on a pain scale, and the fourth patient's family members had called the desk three times in five minutes stating they needed to see me "right now."

I had not even listened to report yet so I didn't know the background or diagnosis of my assigned patients, so I just "flew by the seat of my pants," as the saying goes.

One great thing about nursing is teamwork. If a co-worker needs help with a patient, everyone is right there to help no matter what the circumstance. I have seen two nurses be at odds over something petty and then work side by side in harmony while taking care of a patient. This situation was no exception.

Once I called for help, my peers were there in an instant. We assessed the situation and prioritized the patients. I went to the one with chest pain while another nurse checked on the little confused lady, and still another treated the man with the abnormal heart rhythm.

Finally, I asked a peer to check with the family who was calling out to see if she could help them. It turned out they had a question about a test scheduled for their loved one that day, and, at the time, this was not a priority for me. My patient with chest pain was having a heart attack, so I was busy getting him where he needed to be.

When I finally got him to the cath lab and in the hands of a cardiologist, I checked in on my other patients. My peers had taken care of the emergent situations, but I was now way behind on my day. I knew I had to go listen to a report and get my meds passed, but I thought I better go stick my head in each room to introduce myself and explain the situation.

As I crossed the doorway of the fourth patient, the family member jumped up and began raising her voice at me before I could speak. I tried to explain as best I could the confusion of the morning, but she would not hear it.

When the staff person went in that morning and she asked about the test, she naturally expected someone to respond to her.

"I asked about the time of the test because I have to adjust my work schedule in order to be here with him, and no one ever got back to me. Do you understand my frustration?" she said with a cracked voice. "I needed to know and no one seemed to care one way or the other."

I tried again to explain, but I knew it was not going to make a difference. She was angry and nothing I said could make it better. I apologized again and went out to find out the time of the test.

"Please don't tell me that," I said to the technician on the other line. This wasn't good news.

"That's the best I can do," she said. "Our schedule is packed and since he is an in-patient, we will work him in when we can."

I walked down the hall slowly; anticipating how I was going to tell this lady that her husband was "on call" to CT scan because they had to "work him in" today. The out-patient and the critical ill had priority and when they had an opening, they could get him down within minutes. I realized the logic of this, but how in the world could I explain it to her?

The reaction was as I expected and she went to my charge nurse and reported me as "negligent." Fortunately, my manager knew how my day had started and supported me in this situation, but it didn't make me feel any better. I lived that frustration not so long ago as I hung over the desk at the nurses' station looking for Rob so I knew from where it came, but couldn't she just try to understand my position in all this?

As I headed toward the taping room to finally get report on my patients, I glanced at the clock. It was 8:45 a.m. My shift that was supposed to start at 7 a.m. had not even begun and I was already so far behind. It was my third 12 hour day in a row and I had two more this week because I signed up for some extra shifts.

I was stressed and tired, which led me back into my familiar list mode. No lunch for me today. Good thing I threw some protein bars in my purse this morning. Call Adam and tell him I will be late tonight. Make a mental note to get a new pair of shoes because my feet were already killing me. Try to find a way to get the wife of my patient to trust me.

Just then, my pager went off telling me that the daughter of the patient that I sent to cath lab earlier was on the phone and wanted to talk to me about the status of her dad.

"Yep," I said to anyone who would listen. "When I open my hospital, families aren't allowed."

I then smiled and relaxed as I had an instant flashback of my situation with Rob. I knew through my experience that the problem was in the process. Most people don't understand the complicated processes of healthcare, and sometimes we don't do a very good job of explaining them.

I remember when they moved Rob to the ICU and all the aspects of his illness, and the most important thing to my family in our experiences was communication of those details. Once I knew what was going on and the reason for a delay or change in a situation, it was easier to understand and be tolerant of the circumstances.

Knowing what I had to do, I took a deep breath and picked up the phone. "This is Judi. How can I help you?"

Chapter 8
Arms and Legs

*H*ave you ever seen an autopsy? I had the opportunity to observe one during my nursing school clinical rotation, and it was something I will never forget. After the shock of seeing the physical aspect of the situation, I settled down and really used it as a learning experience.

The thing that amazed me the most was how identical we all are on the inside. If we could slide a camera down inside of each one of us, we would not be able to distinguish one human being from another.

We have no problem taking organs from one person and placing them anonymously into another. We donate and receive blood with no thought of where it has been or where it is going. Why then, are some people so quick to judge another on the external differences they see?

Fortunately, bedside nurses encounter many of those differences in their patients on a daily basis, and helping them with their physical and cultural challenges becomes second nature to them.

Nurses not only have to multi-task and critically think about the medical aspect of their patients but also manage the sheer logistics of day to day functioning during these stressful circumstances. This is what

I didn't learn, or at least understand, in nursing school but soon discovered during on-the-job training.

I'll never forget this particular Tuesday morning as I went in to introduce myself to my patients. I had finally settled into a semi-normal routine and felt comfortable with my skills. I had four patients assigned to me this day, and as I entered my first semi private room, I stopped abruptly.

Between two of my patients, they only had one leg. One was a double amputee, and the other was missing his left limb. I had never come across this type of situation before, so I was taken back for a moment.

I nervously told them I would be their nurse today and quickly left the room. As I tried to gather my thoughts and figure out how I was going to maneuver around this situation, I entered my next room.

This man was from Bosnia. He had come to the United States to escape his war-torn country but did not speak English. A local church had sponsored his family, and a few months after they arrived, he suffered a heart attack. I smiled and tried to communicate with him in my awkward ways; flailing my hands and speaking loudly and deliberately. He just kept nodding his head yes, having absolutely no idea what I was saying.

As I slowly backed out of the room, I bumped into another nurse. She was standing there with her hands on her hips and laughing softly.

"He isn't deaf, Judi; he just doesn't speak English." She had heard my one way conversation out in the hallway and was amused by my communication disaster.

"I have two patients who together have one leg, and another who speaks a different language. I haven't even seen my last patient yet and I don't know what to do." She could hear the stress in my voice.

"You go see your other patient and then tell the charge nurse you need an interpreter. I have something I need to do now, but I will meet you in room 7006 in ten minutes. I had that room the other day, and I know that bed one has a wheelchair and bed two has prosthesis. I will help you get them up. They are nice guys and pretty self-sufficient once we get them to their point of safety. Oh, and by the way, they are good roommates for each other. Bed two has a pretty nasty ulcer on his good limb and the chances of him losing his second leg are high. Seeing his roommate is helping him through example. We assigned them to the same room for this purpose."

She patted my back, walked down the hall, and disappeared into a patient's room. I could hear her talking and laughing easily with her patient, and I realized I had so much to learn.

Over the short time I had been working as a bedside nurse, I thought I had the hands-on care pretty much down pat. There were a few skills I still struggled with, but overall, I was feeling okay when I came to work.

I smiled as I remembered when I first became a nurse and wasn't very good at starting IVs. I tried and tried but never could perfect it like some of my co-workers. I went to the experts on the unit and asked for tips, but I really struggled with it. I hated hurting people but my peers were getting tired of me asking them to "look at these veins" for me.

On top of all that, patients would often say, "you have one chance to stick me." Nothing like adding more pressure when you were doing the very best that you could do. I would pray every day while going to work, "Please don't let me have to start any IVs today," but usually I ended up with one or two a shift.

Now I was over that and getting comfortable with those types of things, but these extraneous "outside the box" factors were going to take some time for me to master.

I had many thoughts in this short moment. I realized not only how non-judgmental nurses have to be to work in this field, but how much diversity comes into play in healthcare.

Every patient presents with a different race, color, creed, culture, disability, family situation, and belief system, and "invisible suitcase," to mention a few. Not only is it the expectation that the health needs of people will be addressed but all of these pertinent things as well.

It is second nature to nurses; never blinking an eye at some of the circumstances they see but, instead, just figuring it out one patient at a time. It was an amazing discovery to me.

My attention was also drawn to her description of my patients. Room 7006. Bed one. Bed two. I immediately thought of Rob and his room number name identification and being labeled "the code" in the ER. At the time, it seemed so impersonal.

Anita was an excellent nurse and her calling patients by their room number did not influence her quality of care. Sometimes an assignment will include discharges and admissions throughout the day and a nurse will have contact with seven or eight patients in a shift.

Many times, it is literally impossible to remember all the information, so designation by room number or diagnosis is an organizational skill, not an insult. I thought back to Rob's illness and knew I could not have understood that during such a stressful time.

I made a mental note to remember that it might be okay to do that with my peers, but it was not acceptable for patients or families to hear. Wow! So many things to balance in addition to the medical information I needed to know.

As I turned to head down the hall, another nurse passed me carrying a water pitcher. She smiled and said hello as she passed me to go to the kitchen, and I thought about still another aspect of this role.

I witnessed this same nurse the day before providing emergency care to a patient in need, and now here she was filling a water pitcher.

This thing called nursing began as a primitive hand maiden job. The early pioneers not only provided basic care for patients; they also kept coal in the furnaces for heat, cooked the meals and served them, cleaned the rooms and scrubbed the floors, and gave up their chairs when physicians entered the room.

Now, the medical knowledge and skills are complicated, the responsibility vast, and the diversity of the patient population complex, but the basic care remains most important.

The same nurse who saves lives also fills water pitchers and gets warm blankets. The same nurse who sits at the bedside in the middle of the night holding hands and listening to stories also listens to lung sounds and assesses medical emergencies. The professional nurse and the nurturer all wrapped into one.

I completed my rounds, contacted an interpreter, and we got the guys up out of bed. I learned how to transfer a man with no legs without hurting my back. I discovered how to strap on an artificial leg, and how to communicate important information to someone who doesn't speak my language.

But Anita and my patients taught me so much more that day. Not just the "how-to" maneuvers of what was needed, but how important unconditional acceptance of each other is in healthcare.

Looking at each patient as an individual with specific as well as basic needs is just as important as the medical care provided. And no matter how different on the outside, our internal needs are all the same.

Not only did I learn something more important than critical pathways and test results, but my patients learned something about me as well. I was a person with needs and fears just like them. The goodness in them saw the goodness in me.

When I explained that I had never encountered this particular situation before, the two men and Anita showed me just what to do and how to do it correctly. When the interpreter came, I asked him to explain to my patient that I was new at this, but with his help, we would make sure he received excellent care. I asked about his family and told him about mine. He smiled and nodded again, but this time I knew he understood what I was saying.

The next day, his wife brought in a Bosnian dish for me to take home and share with Adam and a beautiful bound journal she had hand-made.

"Hvala mnogo," I said. I had no idea if it was the correct translation for "thank you," but I gave it a try. I had asked the interpreter for a few words to learn to make him feel more comfortable, and that was one he taught me.

She laughed as she looked at her husband, and I knew I had probably said it wrong. But it didn't matter. We understood each other on that deeper level as one human being to another without the interference of words. I love this job.

Chapter 9

Lunch and Learn

Consider this: Do you work, eat, and socialize all in the same space? Probably not. If you are a nurse, however, it is the norm rather than the exception.

When hospital nurses go to work, they usually go to a specific home unit. Their patient assignment will be a certain group of patients on that unit, and they are the caregiver for the duration of their shift. There is a nurses' station that is sort of a "command center" for the functioning of the unit, and this is a place for staff to gather and exchange information.

Because of the nature of the work, any social conversation or break time that takes place occurs directly inside the unit. Normally, no one leaves because patient care is ongoing.

There is usually a lunch room available, but sometimes it is difficult to take a break and get away for any period of time. The phone rings or pager goes off when there is a need, and many times that is in the middle of a bite of food.

Countless meals are skipped or discarded because of the necessity of being available for any emergency. Usually food is grabbed on the go and eaten at the desk while catching up on charting.

Sometimes, however, there is an opportunity to sit down and eat at a regular pace. When that happened, I would always go in and tell my patients I was leaving the floor for a few minutes and to see if I could do anything for them before I left. It's funny, I could tell that many of them did not like the fact that I was actually going to lunch.

I was not sure of the reason, but it seemed they thought I was putting my needs above theirs, and they had so many needs right then. I was the security to get help if they needed it. It seemed strange to me at the time since there were always other staff available to cover if needed.

"Everyone has to eat, for heaven's sake," I would think to myself. "Especially during a twelve-hour shift."

Then I remembered my "invisible suitcase" theory. I tried to think what they might be carrying around in their baggage and usually just stayed on the unit and watched my own patients.

Socialization is also a vital part of everyone's work life, but normally there is a time and a place for that to occur. Having fun at work is a part of the norm for other employees, but this is also a little different in a hospital.

Trying to celebrate birthdays and weddings in the background while conducting healthcare business is a balancing act, and sometimes impossible to accomplish. Discussions of relationships gone awry and kids soccer games occur in the same work space as the serious medical conversations and procedures, and this can cause some misconceptions from the patient's and the family member's point of view.

One day in early March, I was anxious to talk to my friend Oris. Jeff had graduated from college and moved to the west coast for graduate school. Adam was progressing well through school and back to playing some sports. I had been so preoccupied with completing my education and trying to get re-established as a single person while dealing with all the grief, I never gave much thought to a social life of the dating kind.

Adam and I had been attending a support group called Fernside, a group for children who had lost a parent. While the kids were in their gathering place, the parents would meet in another room and talk about the issues we had in common.

At one of the Monday night meetings, I looked across the room, and for the first time, thought, "My goodness, that man is handsome!" The reaction was instantaneous as my eyes filled up with tears, and I immediately excused myself from the room.

"How dare you," I thought to myself as I leaned across the sink and glanced up into the mirror. The thought of being with another man was nauseating, almost feeling like adultery and a betrayal of Rob.

I pulled myself together long enough to get to my car, but cried all the way home that evening. It was so hard to move forward all alone, and I missed his presence in my life so much. I did everything I could to put this out of my mind, but, despite all the efforts, the attraction remained.

Meeting after meeting, I found my eyes drawn to his side of the room, and when our eyes met, he would smile at me. Four weeks later, he asked me out on a date.

I don't really remember what I said or how I acted, although I was sure it was something silly, but I do remember I said "yes." It was this coming weekend and I needed some advice.

Dating as an adult was foreign to me, and I wanted to talk to Oris about it. Plus, it was just fun to plan, and I hadn't had fun in a very long time.

I finally touched base with her about 11 a.m. in the hallway.

"I need to talk to you," I said giggling like a teenage girl.

She could tell by my expression this wasn't work related, so we pulled up two chairs at the workstation and talked for a few minutes.

I told her the whole story of how this came to be. His wife had died about a year ago, and he had three kids he was raising alone. He was coming over Friday evening to pick me up and go to dinner.

"I'll pick the restaurant and you pick the movie," he said on the phone the night before.

"What do I wear? What do I order? I don't know if I can eat in front of another man! What movie should we see? Do I invite him in afterwards? Oh my God, what am I doing?"

She was laughing at me and with me, and it was a wonderful minute of friendship and fellowship. I missed having a social life, and she had become a good friend at work.

As we were talking, I received a call that my patient wanted to see me regarding his medication list. I had asked his wife to bring it in since he didn't know what medications he was taking at home, and he called to say she was here now and had that information with her.

Knowing this wasn't an emergency, we took a minute to finish our conversation and a big friendly hug, and I went into his room. I smiled, introduced myself to her, and thanked her for bringing in the information, but I could sense something was wrong.

"If you weren't out there talking about your dating life instead of in here helping me like you are paid to do, this could have been settled before now."

"I'm sorry?" I asked as a question, not quite catching on to his insinuation.

"I could hear you out there laughing and talking about a date while I am in here sick and needing help. I can't believe they pay you to sit and gossip. No wonder health care costs so much!"

My initial reaction was devastation. I was so embarrassed that a patient heard me in the hall talking about my upcoming Friday night date. But then my frustration took over. Where was I supposed to have a conversation with my friend? Patient care was not affected by this innocent friendship exchange so why did it matter so much to him?

I apologized and fixed the situation at hand, but the thoughts continued to haunt me.

I went home that night and told Adam the story. Without even looking up from the science book in front of him, he said,

"It would make me mad too. I remember hearing people laughing and talking when Rob (yes, he called him Rob, but that story is for another time) was in the ICU and I wanted to yell at them and say "my dad is sick. Quit laughing."

I was speechless. Out of the mouth of babes! But I continued.

"So, I am not supposed to talk all day long? Where do I have a conversation with my friends?"

"I don't know. That's for you to figure out." He continued to do his homework, and I sat in silence.

Over the next few days, I watched and listened to the conversations conducted on the unit. The change of shifts were especially noisy as we crossed paths with our peers who worked opposite us, but it was a short time period because most wanted to get on with their work or get home.

There was some laughing and talking throughout the day but it didn't seem especially loud. Some would receive personal calls on their phones but they were short and to the point.

I even watched people interact with each other in different work environments like the grocery store or the bank. Everyone there was discussing their personal stories, and the customer didn't seem to be affected. I knew a hospital was a different environment, but how do we balance the staff's needs with those of our patients and families? We don't laugh or talk during emergencies, so why did this particular situation have such a strong emotional impact on my patient?

It upset him enough that he mentioned it on a customer service survey he returned after he was discharged. Try explaining that to your manager!

I thought of Adam's observation along with the memory of the conversation I overheard in the ER when Rob died, and decided to keep this in mind whenever I conducted a personal conversation at work.

The weekend came and went, and my date was a disaster. Oris anxiously approached me the following week and asked for all the details.

"I want to hear all about it," she said.

I took her by the arm and whispered, "Oh, it was not good. I have a lot to tell you. Let's go to the lounge for just a minute so we can talk in private."

"I can't. I am pretty busy but we will catch up later."

It took us two days to finally connect, but that was just the nature of the situation. The complexity of socialization at work and the fragility of patients were made apparent to me that day, but it wasn't until much later that I finally completely understood it.

Chapter 10
The Unforgettable Ones

I was in an airplane last week, and the weather was cool and cloudy. As we bounced around in the air and the fasten-seat-belt sign came on, the pilot announced he was going to move up above the clouds to find a smoother pathway.

"It will be rough for a minute or two," he said, "but we will be fine once we reach a higher elevation."

We began a steady rough climb, but as we broke through the cloud formation, the sun was there to greet us and the ride immediately became even and steady. Some passengers even broke out into a spontaneous applause.

I thought of a few of my patients, and this scenario reminded me of them. When some people are admitted to the hospital, they go into what I call "sick mode." Even after having surgery and improving their physical status, they remain in an emotionally sick state.

The perception of being sick is just as strong as the physical illness itself, and some patients cannot overcome that hurdle. They stay below the clouds and continue on a turbulent pathway, just like the low flying aircraft I was in that day.

As a nurse, caring for these patients can be very frustrating. Many don't want to get out of bed and expect the staff to do everything for them. I even had one man demand I hold the cup of water while he took a sip when there was no physical reason he couldn't do it himself.

"I am sick and that is your job," he said when I questioned why I should feed him.

"You are not sick, and you are physically capable of holding your own cup. Who is going to hold it for you when you get home?" I asked teasingly.

"My wife," he answered abruptly.

I rolled my eyes and reached for the cup. "My job is to help you get back to your normal life and you aren't allowing me to do that," I tried to explain. As we were talking, his wife arrived and entered the room.

He immediately blurted out, "Thank goodness you are here. She won't even hold this cup for me so I can take a sip of water, and I am really thirsty."

Before I could even respond, she ran over to the bedside and grabbed the cup. As she placed the straw in his mouth, she rubbed his forehead and said, "It's okay honey. I'm here now."

He curled up in bed like a small child and drank his water without moving a muscle.

I wanted to tell them the importance of returning to a normal routine as soon as possible after surgery, but I could see I wasn't going to win this discussion with either one of them.

As I left the room, I remembered Rob and his attitude after his heart transplant. Just like this wife, I also tried to do everything I could for him in those early post op days. I was just so happy he had lived through the surgery and I wanted to feel like I was doing something for him.

"I am not an invalid, Judi. I can feed myself. I have a new heart, not a new arm," he would say as he laughed out loud. No sick mode for him.

The doctor said it was one of the reasons he recovered so quickly. Attitude is everything during physical convalescence, and Rob chose to fly above the clouds and take the smooth route. This is where the sun still shines even in the darkest storms.

Not everyone chooses to live in that mindset, so balancing personality with freedom of choice makes for some interesting interactions. Each day, someone makes a decision that we may or may not agree with, but acceptance is part of the job.

Being an advocate for a patient is second nature to a nurse, but watching someone make bad choices and not being able to do anything about it is hard. Harry is the patient who immediately comes to mind when discussing bad choices.

He is what we in healthcare call a "frequent flyer." I've had several under my care over the years, but Harry stands out above the rest.

Many patients do not heed the life style changes needed to improve their health status after a medical diagnosis so they return to the hospital on a regular basis. They continue to smoke, drink, and eat unhealthy foods with no intention of altering any habits.

"I am not giving up anything," one diabetic woman told me. "When I need something fixed, I'll just come in here and let you do that. That's why you are here."

It becomes very discouraging to a nurse whose goal is to have good quality outcomes. Teaching patients how to take control of their own health is one of the most fulfilling roles of nursing.

Over the course of four years, Harry was a patient on our unit 23 times. He had nineteen stents placed in his heart in addition to two open heart surgeries. "The bionic man," was a term of endearment staff used to describe him.

"I want a wing of the hospital named after me when I am gone," he once announced as he was being discharged. "See you next time!"

He would throw one hand up in the air to say goodbye while reaching in his pocket with the other for a cigarette to light as soon as he hit the door. Although he was a nice man and made staff laugh, it was difficult to provide the care he required. Each time he went home, I wondered if we would see him again.

It may sound a little strange, but when a nurse sees an obituary of a former patient in the paper, it is brought in and shared with the other staff. Discussions about the last admission and thoughts about the family are topics of conversation throughout the day. Because nurses play such an important part in their lives during the illness, it seems only natural to share thoughts about them in their death.

A veil of sadness lingers in the air. Loss of a patient, either in or outside the hospital, affects everyone on the unit. We may call patients by their room number or diagnosis, but in our hearts, we know them all by name.

I have not yet seen anything written in the newspaper about Harry. For as exasperating and challenging patient as he is, I will breathe a sigh of relief when I see his name appear once again on the admission board.

Dealing with life and death on a daily basis is out of the ordinary for most people but common for nurses. We count on each other to share our stories because the majority of non-medical people really don't understand them. This thing called the conflict of caring is reality.

When a nurse is scheduled to leave work at 7:30 p.m., but doesn't get out until 9 p.m., it is usually because something is going on, and it is not possible to leave.

When I am late for functions or have to cancel appointments because of staying late at work, I ask, "would you want me to leave if it was your mother?" Usually that gets me off the hook.

We can be in the midst of a code blue or have our hands in some weeping wound, and then clean up and grab a bite to eat together. It is a safe environment to talk about the professional and personal aspects of life that others can't appreciate.

We not only share the lives of our patients but also the lives of each other. Some stories are so bizarre that they are passed down over the years to the new staff members. Ruth's story is a prime example.

One February evening, the code light went off on our unit. As I entered the room, I saw them performing CPR on a fragile elderly lady.

"What happened?" I asked Shirley.

"She went out when I was walking her back from the bathroom," she whispered. "Her family just left a few minutes ago. I am trying to find them because they were having a discussion about her code status. I am not sure we should be doing this."

I recognized the anxiety in her voice. It is always necessary to know the wishes of patients during these situations because, if we don't know, we have to resuscitate.

Several medications and one shock had already been given to the patient when the family arrived. They told us to stop the code because an honest conversation had taken place earlier with their mom and she told them she did not want any of this.

As they went to the chapel to say a prayer for Ruth, they heard the code light go up and just knew it was her.

"She said she was ready," her daughter whispered. The activity around Ruth came to a stop, and the staff slowly left the room.

As the family waited, three of us went in to clean up and prepare the body. When we do post mortem care, there is a solemn atmosphere in the room. If we talk, it is softly and respectfully.

I was packing up the belongings because that was still such a vivid memory for me, and Shirley was wiping Ruth's face. All of a sudden, "Aghhhh," we heard come from Ruth. All three of us froze in place. We watched and listened, and nothing happened.

Then again, "aghhhh." I ran out into the hallway and grabbed the resident.

"She is making a noise! She is breathing!"

The doctor came in and listened with his stethoscope. While he was in there, Ruth did another sporadic gasp. Then nothing. He continued to listen.

"I believe it is just from all the medications we gave her during the code. Sometimes there is a chemical response and if that is the case, it will slowly subside. Let's finish up here and place her in a private room. This way, the family can have some personal time together and we can continue to monitor her."

I remembered Rob and the cold stark room where he had died. I was not allowed back there until they gave me permission to do so. Because of our unit's family centered care policies, at least Ruth and her family would be comfortable and could take as much time as they needed to be with their loved one and to say their goodbyes. I was glad I worked in a nurturing environment.

Shirley moved Ruth and her family to a nice private room and I headed home for the night. The next day, I was helping to pass breakfast trays and I knocked on the door.

"Hello, breakfast is here," I said as I glanced at the liquids on the tray. "Must have had a procedure," I thought to myself as I noticed there were no solids on it.

"Come in," a voice said. As I entered the room and looked up at the patient, I jumped back in amazement and almost dropped the tray. It was Ruth!

"I've witnessed that reaction all morning," she said laughing at my loss of composure.

"You died!" I blurted out without thinking! She smiled at me.

"That's what they tell me!"

I had to sit down to gather my thoughts and try to understand what just happened. Evidently, her breathing became more and more regular as time went on. They eventually placed her back on the monitor and she began to have a slow steady heart rate.

Within a few hours, Ruth woke up and was able to speak a few words to her daughter.

"It's a miracle!" she exclaimed!

I asked her if she had seen the light or remembered anything that had happened but she said she had no recollection of anything. I told her that Shirley was the one who was wiping her face, and each time her hands touched Ruth, she took that gasping breath. We decided that Shirley must have some healing energy in her hands, or that Ruth still had some purpose to fulfill.

Either way, it was an amazing story, and I hugged her tightly before I left the room. It was the talk of the hospital for several days.

Ruth was discharged five days later. I have no idea what happened to her after she left us, but the story has carried on for years. Shirley still has the reputation of having "healing hands" and I have never witnessed anything remotely like this since then.

Now tell me, how do you go home and begin to share a story like that? We work and play and socialize and love all in the same place and meet some incredible people. And one thing is for sure; despite all the conflicts, nursing is a profession like no other.

Chapter 11
The Passing of Shay

"*T*hank you," she whispered softly, barely moving her dry parched lips. Shay broke my heart. She was a 28-year-old mother of two who was terminally ill.

During her last pregnancy, she had noticed a lump in her breast but it was thought to be an enlarged milk gland. It continued to grow after the birth of her daughter, and eventually she insisted on a mammogram despite her young age.

After all the tests and biopsies were conducted, Shay was diagnosed with stage four breast cancer with metastasis throughout her small fragile body. She was on our telemetry floor because she had a very fast heart rate, and her physician wanted her to be monitored.

One thing that is so satisfying to a nurse is when a patient or family member says "thank you." Appreciation goes a long way during a 12 hour shift or on Christmas day when your kids are at Grandma's and you are at work.

Many times I have said to Jeff and Adam, "Santa comes tomorrow at our house because I have to go take care of the sick people." They always understood and even came with me a few times to visit the patients, but it was still hard to leave them. So when a patient thanked me for helping them or for working on a holiday, it was so very nice.

I still have a drawer filled with all my notes and cards from patients who sent words of thanks and let me know how they were doing. Gratitude is a wonderful thing to a nurse but can be overwhelming at the same time.

"You don't have to keep thanking me, Shay. It is an honor to care for you," I said as I brought her some juice.

"I just want you to know I appreciate not only your physical care of me, but your emotional and personal support as well," she said slowly in between breaths.

I sat down beside her and held her hand. She was so frightened. The day before, I had spent almost an hour sitting and talking with her. Well, actually I did more listening than talking.

Her son was two and her daughter six months, and she worried about what would happen to them after she was gone. Her husband was in denial, not being able to grasp the seriousness of the situation, and her mother was too sick to raise them. We discussed so many personal things with each other, and the bond between us was strong.

In nursing school we are taught the difference between empathy and sympathy and all the textbook ways to handle emotional situations, but when you are in the middle of someone's life and death, it is hard to function within those parameters.

Nurses get involved in the lives of their patients. That's just the way it is. They hold weddings, go to funerals, have anniversary parties in hospital rooms, and bring a touch of personal life to a professional setting when the need arises.

One patient was on our unit for almost eight months. During the holidays, we decided to decorate his room to cheer him up. Someone brought in a small Christmas tree and another some garland and lights.

By the time we were finished, it was a Christmas showcase, and he was so thrilled. Every visitor who came to see him heard the story of what his nurses had done for him. It raised his spirits, and I know it helped in eventually getting him well enough to go home.

A few years ago, another patient was too sick to attend his daughter's wedding, so the wedding took place on our unit.

The family came in and decorated the classroom beautifully and furnished the music and the minister. Everyone came to the hospital. The bride walked down our hallway and the staff pushed the hospital bed alongside her so her dad could walk his daughter down the aisle.

It was the most beautiful and emotional wedding I have ever attended. We even had a small reception for them before they went off to the larger one that evening. He was so grateful for what we had done but we were just as happy to be able to do it for him. There wasn't a dry eye on the unit that day.

As his health continued to deteriorate and he realized he wasn't going to be able to go back home, his only request was to "see and feel the sun shine one more time." Once again, a nurse had an idea.

She got an order that allowed us to take him out on our patio in his hospital bed. The family came in and spent the entire afternoon outside in the sun with their loved one. The grandchildren climbed up in the bed with him, and there was laughter and joy that could be felt throughout the unit. The newlyweds were there, and we were all happy to see them and hear about the recent purchase of their new house.

As he came back into his room that evening and said goodbye to his family, he was more relaxed and content than I had ever seen him. Two days later, he went to sleep and never woke up.

The family was so grateful for all we had done, but really we were the fortunate ones. When nurses are able to provide holistic care to their patients and families that is meaningful, they are fulfilled as well. This is how I felt about taking care of Shay.

Ever since high school, Shay had been an avid reader, but she just couldn't concentrate on anything at this point. Whenever I had an extra minute, I went in and read a chapter to her from one of her books, and I would talk about the story. She was so short of breath that she couldn't discuss anything at length but I knew by the way she shook her head and looked at me whether she agreed with my point of view or not.

This day was difficult for her. Out of bed, in bed; lying down or sitting up; nothing seemed to work. I tried rubbing her back and massaging her feet, but her skin was so sensitive to touch, it seemed to hurt her more than it helped. I was frustrated because I wanted so desperately to help her. That is what we do; we fix things for our patients. But this I could not fix.

She even snapped at me at one point and then immediately took my hand and cried.

"It is okay," is all I could think to say.

I stayed about an hour after my shift was over and helped her freshen up. Her husband was bringing the baby in and she wanted to have on a clean gown when she held her. We got her as comfortable as we could in a chair with pillows and a blanket, and combed her hair enough to look "presentable" as she put it.

When her husband came around the corner with that precious little girl, Shay's smile lit up the room. It was my last image of her. I said my goodbyes and went home.

About 11:30 that night, my phone rang. It was the charge nurse telling me Shay had passed away. The visit with her family had gone well, but she had become more and more short of breath after they left.

They told me that before she lost consciousness, she called out my name like she always did when she wanted me to come to her room. When they reminded her that I had gone home for the night, she nodded her head liked she remembered. Within the next few hours, she was gone.

I had never experienced the type of grief and mourning that I felt with the loss of Shay since Rob's death a few years earlier. I sobbed so hard and so long, I wasn't sure I could contain myself. The feelings of guilt overcame me once again; I should have stayed; I could have done more. But in the end, there was nothing else to do for Shay. She was at peace.

I knew from the experience with Rob, that guilt was a toxic emotion and did no one any good. I did not want to start packing up my invisible suitcase again. Guilt made the load so heavy, and Shay would not want that for me anyway.

The funeral was a beautiful reflection of her life, and I spent most of the day in fellowship with her family and friends.

As I left that evening, her mother took me in the den and pointed to a box. "We want you to have these," she said to me. As I bent and opened the cardboard flap, I smiled and hugged her tightly.

"I am so sorry for your loss, Ethel. I loved her too and I will miss her so much."

"We know honey. You are a wonderful nurse. That was obvious the first day you entered her room, but you quickly became more than that to all of us.

You not only cared for her medical needs, but you cared for all of us. You gave us information, you gave us your time, and you gave us your patience and understanding when we acted out. I know this was not easy for you with all you have experienced. That Rob was a lucky man."

As I had gotten to know Shay and her family, I had shared Rob's story with them.

"Yes he was," I whispered and finally released my arms from around her back. "Thank you for the books. I will cherish them."

A flood of emotions emanated through my mind on my trip back home. I reminisced about my life with Rob and the vast emptiness his death brought to all of us. Shay's family had a long road ahead of them and my heart ached as I remembered the pain of that hell. Thinking of

Shay made me smile and cry. She was such a magnificent person and friend.

Why was it that so many of the people I cared about left this earth too soon?

"Because you are a nurse," I said out loud.

I recalled a quote someone gave me when Rob died. "I think not of how unhappy I will be when you are gone; instead, I think of how empty I would be if you had never come."

So many of the people in my life I met because I was a nurse; patients, families, other hospital staff. Personal life and professional life merge as one and it becomes difficult to separate one from the other. We come together each day, not just as a job, but for the purpose of caring for each other.

We meet patients at a point when their life has jumped off track and on to a path they did not chose. We share the most vulnerable and poignant parts of our being with each other and form bonds of closeness like no other profession. No job description I've ever read included the role of love and friendship and caring, but it is a big part of the role of a bedside nurse.

Nursing is such a complicated practice. The scientific foundation and knowledge base is vital to the profession, but the human element is so intertwined, the boundaries are not clear, the conflicts never ending.

Nursing has been accused of not exhibiting all the qualities of a profession because of the lack of cohesiveness between its members.

"Day shift can't even get along with night shift," I once read in an article written by some newspaper reporter.

Maybe that is true and maybe it isn't, but this I know to be real: nurses care about their patients. I've witnessed nurses as teachers, advocates, mediators, information specialists, and many other roles too numerous to mention, all in the name of patient care.

It doesn't mean that they don't make mistakes or act unreasonable at times. It doesn't mean that they don't carry their "invisible suitcase" to work some days filled to the brim; it does not mean that they are perfect.

It does mean that they bring everything they have to the table when they enter a patient's room. They see the best and the worst of people while giving all of their physical, emotional, and spiritual energy to each situation.

Nurses balance the humanistic side of illness with the scientific side of healthcare while trying to meet the needs of many. Administration, management, physicians, families and patients all have expectations of nurses, and sometimes those individual perceptions are different than the whole reality.

I compare it to looking at the Rocky Mountains through a single telescope: you only see a small piece of stark rock; one observation. But when you take away the narrow view and see the whole picture, the vision is spectacular. This is the gift of nursing.

Chapter 12
The Three Minute Mile

*T*here is a term we use at work sometimes; the impossible 5%. This describes some of the patients and families that we interact with on a day to day basis, and, no matter what we do, we can't seem to make them happy.

Sometimes it is so draining on the staff that we rotate the patient assignment each day so no one is in there two days in a row. This keeps the nurses fresh while making sure the quality of care remains in place. Thankfully, it is only a fraction of the people we encounter, while the other 95% are amazing to know. It is a privilege to be a part of people's lives when they demonstrate each day the power of the human spirit.

I truly believe that service to other human beings is the key to a purposeful and successful life and, as a nurse, I not only get to do that on a daily basis, but I get paid to do it as well! Patient care has molded who I am and how I have chosen to aspire to be in my own life.

I watched the little elderly lady who came from a nursing home and had no family to visit her put on her daily make up or "my face" as she called it, because she wanted to look presentable for her doctor.

"Honey, can you give me my lipstick?" she asked smiling at me.

I thought, "I can only hope I can have that much dignity no matter what the circumstances."

I saw the determination in the eyes of the stroke patient who was working with the therapist and one slight improvement in his movement made him surge on past any ability he thought he had.

"My role model for strength," I reflected.

I remembered the couple who were both admitted to our unit because they had become ill at the same time. They had been married for 60 years and were worried about each other, so we placed them in the same room together to ease their concerns.

As I entered the room one evening, I found that they had pushed the beds closer together and were holding hands across the night stand.

"This is the meaning of relationship," I said, and vowed to never settle for anything less.

You see, the other side of bedside nursing is what we receive in return.

One of the most powerful examples of human courage I have ever witnessed occurred over a mere three minute time span on my unit.

We have an annual tradition in our city called the mini heart marathon. It is a walk/run race that thousands of people attend to raise money for the American Heart Association, and, because we specialize in the treatment of heart disease, many of our employees participate in the event.

This particular year, several of the staff on our unit were getting together a team to walk in honor of our patients so they were talking about it at work. One of the patients heard the discussions and mentioned to me that he ran that race every year. He was really depressed that he would miss it this time because of his surgery; He had a chest tube in to keep his lung inflated, and was having a difficult time with his length of stay in the hospital.

Because we encouraged and expected patients to get up and walk every day, there was always one or more out walking in our long hallways. This particular man would walk and walk throughout the day, "trying to stay in shape," he would say.

One day I had an idea; why not have a "mini heart marathon" on the unit with the patients. I posed the suggestion to a few of my peers and we decided to give it a try.

We decorated the halls with signs; "You can do it." "Almost there." "Stamp out heart disease." We put mini mile markers out just like on the real course, and even had a water station.

A start and a finish line were designed, and we asked for and received from the AHA some caps and medals that they were going to be giving out at the official race. Someone donated bananas, and we got a CD of the *Rocky* theme for our music.

The hallways were lined with red helium balloons and some streamers. All the staff participated in the preparation and when we were done, you could feel the excitement on the unit.

Now, all we needed were some patients! We were not sure what kind of response we would get but we were going to invite everyone, no matter their circumstance.

Over the next few days, we asked all the patients and their families to participate. We even invited the media and asked people from all over the hospital to come and line the hallways for encouragement.

With absolutely no idea what to expect, that morning we began the process of gathering the participants. Of our 35 patients, 28 wanted to take part and all of them had family members ready to go as well. Those who felt they could not do it asked to be placed by their doorways in order to watch the event.

Many were in wheelchairs, on oxygen, and had multiple IV pumps with cardiac drips infusing, but they wanted to be a part of the walk.

The staff pushed the wheelchairs and pumps, walked beside those who could go on their own, gave out water at the half way point, and distributed the caps.

Before we began the honorary walk, we thanked everyone for their contribution and told the patients, "This is in honor of you."

As the *Rocky* music began and the patients began walking down the hallway, the local news came and filmed the event.

For the next three minutes, all the forces of the universe came together for one cause. It was a surreal moment in time.

As the walk began and the wheelchairs and carts were rolling side by side, a spontaneous applause began from those lining the hallway. Administrators, nurses, secretaries, and respiratory therapists all came to support the walkers.

The vision of 40-plus people walking or being wheeled in unison with a sea of red caps and IV pumps was overwhelming to witness. The young man who said he had never missed a race was the leader of the pack, but he walked slowly so that all patients could circle the hallway together. The smiles from all the participants were enough to light up the unit, and the patients in the doorways said encouraging words as they passed by.

As they crossed the finish line, bright shiny medals were placed around their neck. Many of them cried as they completed the circle; the circle of life they called it, and told us it was the best experience of their life.

I watched as they walked and I saw scars; chest, leg, arm, abdomen scars from the surgeries they had to help restore and heal their physical body.

But I also saw the emotional scars of illness and surgery being healed by being part of a cause bigger than each individual—the cause of an internal human connectedness that cannot be described in words. There was a spirit of love for our fellow man. Where else can you work and witness a miracle such as this?

The walk lasted a total of three minutes but its effects were timeless. The young man who had not missed a race sends a card every year telling us how grateful he was for what we did and how it has affected his life since then.

Some patients told us the following day that they slept with their medals on because they were so proud to be a part of something so special. One lady confessed she didn't even want to live anymore up to that point, but after participating in the walk, she was motivated to get better. She got well enough to go home, but her family sent a note a few months later telling us she had passed away.

"We displayed her medal at the funeral home," they wrote in their note. "It was her most prized possession."

Nursing is always number one or two in the annual national list of most respected professions. We have earned that respect through hard work, dedication, continual learning, and caring.

One of my family members works for a non-profit organization, and the list of nursing volunteers is in the thousands. To volunteer for a mission means losing work time and paying expenses out of their own pocket, but despite that, the list continues to grow.

Nurses are not just care givers, but also givers of caring. They consider it a privilege to be a part of each individual life they encounter, and share in the joys and heartaches of all their patients and families.

But nurses receive so much more than they give; they receive the gift of human connectedness as experienced in that three minute walk on a step-down unit. The gift of observing the spirit of love at its deepest level. The gift of the bond between a nurse and a patient.

Part Three:
The Patient's View

"The human spirit is stronger than anything that can happen to it."

— C. C. Scott

Chapter 13
The Personal Experience

I had on the pair of scrub pants that had a small yellow stain on the right side. When I had done my laundry the week before, I forgot to check my clothes, and I washed the pants with a vitamin pill still in the pocket. It wasn't bad enough to discard them, so I put them on, making a mental note to see if anyone noticed it.

My shirt was long sleeved and my jacket had a small tear at the left seam. My shoes were a few weeks old but were broken in pretty well, and it was a particularly good hair day. I can recall every detail about the day that would change the rest of my life.

Life had settled into somewhat of a routine for me, and things were going well. Jeff had continued his education and received his PhD. He was working in California as a researcher and recently engaged to Ellen.

Adam had finished college and wanted to follow in his brother's footsteps. He was in a PhD program in California as well and lived about 20 minutes from Jeff.

"It's going to be one coast or the other," he told me, as he was applying to schools.

When he chose a program near Jeff, I have to admit I was happy. If he was going to move away from home, at least he would be near family. In the end, it worked out great for me as I could visit both of them at the same time when I went on vacation.

I had never re-married, although I came close a few times. I had gone back to school for my master's degree and had built a close social network of friends. I stayed busy and continued to grow as a nurse, but the hole in my heart remained.

Grief is a funny thing. You can go through life feeling fairly normal, but the sadness lies right beneath the surface. Sometimes it rears its ugly head and emerges without notice and can knock you back into the depths of sorrow as if the loss had just occurred. I think this affected any relationship I attempted to have, but I have to believe it all worked out for the best.

I was still working on the cardiac floor but was now the manager of the unit. My professional goals did not include a management job, but I did not want someone from outside our hospital to run my floor. I had so much invested in my work environment that, when the opportunity arose, I took on the role.

Success is measured in many ways, but I can only say that life was good; well, at least as good as it could be with Rob gone and the boys grown and living away.

I was always religious about getting my annual health screenings. I saw so many patients who said they had never gone to a doctor until they got sick, and by then their health was already compromised, so I strongly believed in preventative medicine.

I had my mammogram the day after Christmas and everything went as usual. When I received a call to come back and have a repeat film, I didn't think a thing of it. It had happened many times before and I always said I would rather be safe than sorry.

An ultrasound was done after the repeat films, followed by a visit from the physician.

"There are a couple of small areas that were not on your films last year," she said as she placed them in the viewer. "I would like to biopsy them."

She pointed to two small dots on the x ray film and I was surprised to see how little they were. I had to move in closer to actually see them.

"Okay," I said hesitantly, and she could hear the uncertainty in my voice.

Before I could tell her that I was actually pleased that she recognized those tiny differences; that at 4 p.m. in the afternoon she had paid just as much attention to my films as the first films of the day, she continued on.

"Our screening process has become much more sophisticated so we are discovering smaller calcifications, but I want you to know that 85% of all the biopsies we do come back negative."

With reassurance in her voice and a tender touch on my arm, I felt at ease.

"Okay. What do I need to do next?" I asked.

They suggested a stereotactic biopsy. I had heard the term before but wasn't quite sure of the process.

I was taken into a room where I had to lay face down on a table with a hole in it. My left breast was placed down into the hole so the doctor and technician could assess if it was possible to obtain the biopsy this way.

"If the areas of the affected breast can be accessed with the vacuum needle through this process," they explained, "it is better than having to go to the OR and be put to sleep for surgery."

It was a tedious course of action; pushing, pulling, stretching the breast while trying not to move and having my arm above my head, but in the end, it was decided that attempting this method was worth a try.

I got dressed, went to the desk to make an appointment for the biopsy, and went back to work.

Being in the healthcare profession, I understood the logic of the situation. Something doesn't look right, we run tests.

Many times I have gone into a patient's room and explained situations exactly like this.

"Your x-ray revealed an atypical area so we are ordering a CT scan to rule out anything serious." "Your EKG looks abnormal so you are scheduled to go to the cath lab today to see if you have any blockage."

It all seemed so obvious to me. You find something wrong; you check it out and fix it.

"Being upset is understandable, but wouldn't you want to know if something was wrong so you could get it fixed?" I used to think to myself. Now I could experience that question first hand.

I called my sister as soon as I returned to my office. If you would ask either one of us if we were close, we both would say yes, but many times weeks would go by without any contact between us.

I was the oldest; Donna would laugh and call herself the "mistreated middle child," and our youngest sister Jo lived in Washington. Three totally different personalities and lifestyles but forever bonded emotionally.

Being raised in that alcoholic atmosphere had its effect on us and we all handled it differently. I believe it is the reason we all went our separate ways; our invisible baggage was too much to bear at the time, but we eventually figured out a way to be close again. We were all just a phone call away.

Donna listened to my story, and talking about it helped me to sort it all out for myself. Sometimes just saying things out loud puts them into perspective.

"They are just being cautious," she said. "Let me know when it is and I will go with you."

I felt better. Donna always had a way to make everything sound practical and logical. Sometimes when I was sad and lonely, I would call her and complain.

"There are worse things than being single," she would say humorously. "One of them is being married." We would both laugh, and I would immediately cheer up.

My biopsy was scheduled for 8 a.m. We arrived a few minutes early, so we sat in the waiting room and talked. It was nice to catch up and share stories of our kids since they lived out of town. Jeff and Adam were in California; her son had relocated to Colorado.

I was a little nervous, but not too bad, and having Donna there helped to divert my attention.

As the technician came out and called my name, we both stood up. Originally, I had been told she could go back with me, but today that was not the case. "This is just like any other procedure area. Visitors cannot come back into the room, but we will keep your family updated throughout the biopsy."

Our eyes met as we squeezed each other's hand.

"I'll be right here," she said as she sat back down. I went back alone.

The physician was in the room and greeted me warmly when I entered. I had just been in a meeting with him a week earlier and here I was, getting ready to strip down in front of him.

There are positive and negative aspects to getting your medical treatment in the facility in which you work. On one hand, knowing the staff and the surroundings is comforting, yet knowing the staff and the surroundings is personally embarrassing, if you know what I mean.

I remember one situation when I had gone to the gynecologist for my Pap smear on Tuesday and had a conversation about a patient in hallway with the same doctor on Wednesday.

"I wonder what he is thinking," I thought to myself. This situation sparked that same feeling.

I got undressed and into a gown. As my left arm was removed from the opening and I was positioned on the table, I tried to be as accommodating as I could; I wanted to be sure everything went as planned. They used cushions for positioning and blankets to keep me warm.

My left chest was placed down into the opening on the table, and the technician sat down next to me. The breast was then compressed into a special mammography machine, and, using x-rays and a computerized device, the calcified region was determined.

Once they located the areas, the stereo view pictures were taken and the precise placement for the procedure to be successful was transmitted. Typically, a numbing medication is then used, and the biopsy needle is guided to the exact area to obtain the sample. The beauty of this procedure is that there is no surgical incision, and you can go right back to your daily routine.

However, for the next hour, I was placed in multiple positions trying to see if that course of action could be accomplished. Arm up, arm down. My breast was pulled and positioned until I thought I couldn't stand it anymore.

The technician and the doctor talked to each other about the positioning of the breast and the accessibility to the intended areas. They were kind and apologetic to me, and I could hear the frustration in their voices. They just weren't sure they could get a good sample this way.

My mind began processing the situation.

"I want to be sure they can get the right areas; they are so small; try not to move; what if they take a sample and it is not the calcified sections; I don't want to have surgery; I hope they can get it; maybe I should hope they can't get to it so I can have surgery and be sure the biopsy is accurate; I just want to be sure it is the exact area."

I could hear them discussing the situation and I wanted to state my concerns, but I just listened.

"I am so sorry, Judi," the radiologist finally said. "I just don't think we can get a good sample this way. I hate that we put you through all this for nothing, but it was worth a try. Normally, it works well, but your calcifications are located in areas that are difficult to access this way. I don't feel comfortable trying again. I want to be sure we get the exact locations so I recommend we do a surgical biopsy."

I experienced a mixture of emotions, but mostly relief. I agreed with his decision; I wanted to get it right too.

"Okay," I said stoically. I was not looking forward to surgery, but it looked like I had no other choice.

I got dressed and met with the radiologist before I left. I asked for the name of a surgeon and was given a few recommendations.

"Let us know who you chose and we will send the films. Again, I am sorry this didn't work out."

"I would rather be safe than sorry," I responded for the second time. "I appreciate your efforts and concerns." I tried not to sound disappointed.

I knew through experience that not everything goes as planned in medicine. We do our best, but, at the end of the day, you realize nothing in life is perfect. You have to go with the flow and keep a positive attitude.

I walked out to meet my sister and told her the news. We both sat in silence for a few minutes, trying to gather our thoughts. Then she made a few phone calls. My emotions were getting the best of me and I didn't want to lose control in the middle of the medical office building.

She saw the somber look on my face, and came over and linked her arm through mine

"Let's go find a surgeon," she said, as we headed toward the elevators.

Chapter 14

The Simple Truth

*T*hink about this: How would you like it if someone came in and took you out of your house and placed you into a group home; took away your clothes and told you what to wear; informed you when and what you were going to eat, who and when others could come visit with you, and something as simple as water was available only if someone brought it to you? Well, this is what it feels like to be a patient.

Loss of control of your day-to-day living is not easy; if anyone else tried to impose these restrictions on any of us, we would protest loudly. But when you enter the hospital as a patient, it is the norm.

Of course, everyone knows there has to be a process in place during admission to a hospital; how haphazard it would be if everyone did their own thing. But looking from the outside in, the process seemed to be centered more toward the institutional needs than the patient's.

Being a nurse, I needed the process in order to be organized and do my job, but as a patient, it amplified the stress of a medical situation.

It also automatically placed some of the patients into that "sick mode" mentality. No wonder patients frequently told me they "just wanted to go home," and families would add, "She is not normally like this," when their loved one was acting out.

I was lying on the stretcher in the same day surgery area trying to come to terms with the present situation. After meeting with the surgeon, I felt pretty good. He had reiterated the fact that most biopsies are negative, and the screenings are so precise now that many things are seen on film that would not have been detected a few years ago. Yet, I was still going for surgery and I have to admit, I was scared.

Earlier in the morning, I had to report to the Breast Center for something called needle localization. It is a procedure that is done prior to surgery to isolate the areas that needed to be removed.

Since my abnormal areas were so small, they could not be felt. The surgeon would have no way to know where the calcifications were, so they had to be identified through the placement of guide wires.

A biopsy mammogram was done for location, and then a needle was placed right next to the affected areas. When the radiologist was sure it was in the right place, the needle was withdrawn, and a small wire was left behind to guide the surgeon to the specific area.

This took about 45 minutes, and, after the wires were taped down, we walked across the driveway to the same day surgery area for the actual biopsy.

There was always a technician by my side during the entire procedure. They were kind and attentive, but it was so embarrassing to expose my chest in front of co-workers, no matter the circumstances. They did not make me feel that way; it was an internal self-consciousness, and I was glad when it was over.

Everyone kept telling me not to worry; it was part of their job, but the problem was, it was part of my job as well. I did not like this side of the bedrail, and I wanted to get back to my control of the situation.

The same day surgery area was bright and cheerful. I was given a patient gown that was difficult to keep closed in the back, and I had to watch that I did not snag those valuable wires. It took two sticks to get the IV in my arm, and I now knew why patients would tell me that they would only give me one chance to get it in; it hurt.

Knowing I would be intubated and have my breathing dependent on someone else made me a little nervous.

"Knowing your surgeon is valuable information, but more importantly, you better be finding out who your anesthesiologist is," my nursing instructor would jokingly say in class.

Well, I had just met him, and he had my information on an index card. He seemed nice, but I worried that I might have forgotten to tell him something important.

My sister was with me and that support was comforting. Even though our conversation was mostly small talk to pass the time, I was so happy she was there.

I thought of all those patients that I had sent to surgery in the past that had no one with them, and it made me sad. I would see the doctor's note stating that there was no one available to talk with after surgery, so I would try to make it a point to ask the patient if there was anyone they wanted me to call when they returned to their room. Knowing I had someone in the waiting room who would talk to the surgeon was comforting to me.

As we talked, I glanced around the room and saw my clothes folded up and stacked in a plastic bag. I thought of Rob and asked Donna if she would keep my belongings with her.

"I'm afraid they will get lost, and I really like that top," I explained. Really, I just wanted them with someone who personally cared about me and my things.

As we waited, I watched the nurses. I knew many of them and several others stopped in to say hello. I could hear the chatter in the hall and some of the conversations with other patients.

I knew the routine; so many forms and computer work to do; arm band for identification and signatures for consent for surgery. It almost seemed like an assembly plant. I could hear the anesthesiologist go room to room saying the same things and asking the same questions.

As a nurse, it was reassuring to me to hear them talk to our patients, knowing they were collecting the correct and comprehensive information, but as a patient, it now seemed somewhat impersonal.

Were we all alike? How can they tell one of us from another in that sterile operating room? Was I just a breast and my next door neighbor a hip?

I remember hearing a woman who came to our workplace a few years ago as a motivational speaker. Her name was Emory Austin. She talked about her experience after having a mastectomy, and how she also worried about being just a statistic.

"I didn't want to be known as just a diagnosis or a room number to my doctor," she explained to us." "I wanted to have a name."

Her desire to be known as an individual led her to have a tee shirt made for her surgeon that said, "One of America's top ten breast men." Why? She wanted him to remember who she was.

She followed up with the fact that, although she worried that he might think it was silly, her desire to be known as a person was more than her concern about making a fool of herself, so she did it anyway.

After she had given him the shirt, she was surprised by his response; "You did that just for me?" he asked surprisingly.

You see, no matter our status or income level, we all just want to be thought of as an individual with our own personal attributes and characteristics. Our own special story. A person; not a body part, or a room number, or a job description.

My thoughts were interrupted when the third person entered my room and asked me which breast was being biopsied and if I had any allergies. My sister listened in silence, but after they left, she questioned the competency of the system.

"Does the right hand know what the left hand is doing?" she inquired as she stood up and straightened my blanket. I could tell she was nervous too.

"It's okay," I said. "It is a requirement, and anyone who has anything to do with this surgery will ask the same thing."

But her question made sense to me. From the patient's and family's point of view, it did seem like none of the information was being shared. I only knew the routine because I had done it so many times. Maybe if it was explained to patients that many people were going to ask the same questions and that safety was the reason for it, there would be a little less stress for them.

As I filed it under "something to remember when sending a patient to surgery" in my mind, the nurse came in and announced, "They are ready for you. I have your pre-op medications."

I woke up in the recovery area in more pain than I anticipated.

"Did it go okay?" I asked the nurse sitting next to me as soon as my eyes opened.

"Yes, they were able to get a good biopsy of both sites," she said smiling. I sighed with relief. Finally I could get this behind me and get back to normal. "I will bring your family back now that you are awake," she said as she paged the volunteer.

I was glad the hospital had a family-centered care culture that included the recovery area. They allowed the family to come back and visit for a few minutes while a patient was recovering, and this is is beneficial for everyone. The patient feels better, the family member's anxiety level is reduced, and staff satisfaction improves.

Donna pulled up a chair and sat beside me.

"I spoke with your surgeon," she began. "He thought everything looked pretty good. He was able to get to both areas and the results will be back in a few days. We will need to celebrate when you feel better."

After a glass of juice and my discharge instructions, I was allowed to go home. It felt good to be back in my own clothes and in my own environment. The pain medicine helped me to sleep that night but the next morning, the surgical site continued to throb.

I went into work later that morning and called the surgeon to see what I could do for the pain. I went over to his office and, as he took off the dressing, I looked at my stitches. The breast was twice the size of the other one and the skin was red and taut.

"You have a hematoma," he said while pressing on a large knot in the lower half of my chest. "You did stop taking the aspirin like you were instructed to do before surgery, didn't you?" he asked.

"Yes. I stopped a week before the surgery date," I explained.

"Well," he hesitated, "we can go back in and remove the clot, or you can apply some heat and it will eventually reabsorb. It may take a while though."

"I will use the heat," I responded quickly. "No more surgery."

I finished the work day as best I could and then went home and cried from the pain.

"All of this just for some artifact on a film," I said to myself. Pain makes things seem worse than they really are.

With each passing day, the knot got harder and harder. It was so tender that when I drove over a bump in the road, I would have to support my chest with my arm. Any movement was painful and clothes were irritating to the touch.

I had to laugh though. The bruising extended over and under my arm and down my abdomen; I looked like I had been in a bar fight and lost, and the swelling made it appear as though I had gotten a one-sided breast implant.

I continued to work and go about my normal routine, using the heat application as often as I could, knowing this would all soon be over.

A few days later, I was at my desk working on payroll when my phone rang. It was a busy day, and I had not had lunch yet.

"Mrs. Schofield?" the voice on the other end said.

"Yes," I answered as I continued to do computer work. Mulit-tasking is a normal part of the day for a nurse, even if it is a nurse working in an office.

"This is Doctor Preston."

"Oh yes," I replied as I stopped what I was doing to concentrate on our conversation.

"We got your biopsy back and….. It showed a little cancer." My mind came to a stop, my eyes blurred, and my heart skipped a beat.

"What?" I asked like I had misunderstood what he had said.

"One of your biopsies came back benign but the other one had some cancer in it. It was very small; in fact all the margins around the cancer site were clear so we don't have to take out anymore tissue because we got it all. I think all you will need is a little radiation to the site, but you will have to find a medical oncologist to manage this for you. We radiate the site of the biopsy just to be sure we didn't miss a cell or two during the surgical process. Why don't you come in tomorrow and we can talk about this in more detail in the office?"

"What time?" Was all I could think to say in response.

The word "cancer" changes everything in your life from that moment on. I could not wrap my thinking around it. What did it mean for me? And, a LITTLE cancer?! Is that like a little pregnant?

I hung up the phone and sat in place. Having a head-on collision with my mortality was staggering, and I wasn't sure what to do next.

"Cancer," I said out loud to no one. "Who do I tell first? What do I say? He said it was small. Maybe it is nothing. Can cancer of any size be nothing?"

The phone rang but I ignored it. I didn't want to conduct business; I had cancer, for goodness sake. Did they not get it?

I realized how irrational my thoughts were and decided to call my sister. She kept me grounded and I needed that right now. She listened to my story and gave me the "at least" version. At least it was small; at least they found it early; at least it was only radiation.

She began to tell me the stories of women she knew that had breast cancer years ago and were now doing great…one was a 25-year survivor. It would be alright.

I deeply appreciated her gallant efforts to make me feel better, but until you are the one with the disease, you do not understand the personal impact of it all.

I remembered as I stood by Rob's coffin with two young children and people would say things to try to make sense of this senseless situation.

"When God closes one door, he opens another," and, "Rob would want you to be strong," they would say as they passed by.

I knew in my heart that every word was meant to help me, but at the time, what I really wanted to say was, "that is the stupidest thing I have ever heard. What the hell does that even mean? What does a closed door have to do with the death of a young husband and father? How do you know what Rob would want for me?"

That was how I felt again. I didn't want to hear "at least" right now. I wanted to curse and scream and throw things. That seemed more logical during this most illogical time.

I knew I had to call my sons. Taking a deep breath, I dialed the numbers and made sure I spoke in an upbeat fashion and tried to make it sound nothing more than a minor inconvenience.

Being the scientist, Jeff wanted a copy of the pathology report and Adam said he was sure everything would be fine. I think it was such a surprise to them because I was just never sick. I hadn't missed a day of work or school in years and had even run a marathon a few years earlier with a fractured kneecap. I was the caregiver, not the care receiver.

I remembered when the boys were very young and I worried about being the only parent. Bargaining with the heavens was a daily occurrence.

"Dear God, please let me live long enough to raise my sons. They cannot be orphans; please God. Please give me enough time to get them up and out on their own."

That time had now come and gone, but at the present moment, I wanted to renegotiate that time line. I wasn't ready to go anywhere just yet.

As I told my diagnosis to a few of my close friends at work, I felt bad for them. They did not know what to say and I could sense their uneasiness. I found myself comforting them and telling them I was sure "everything would be fine." I used all the "at least" versions I could remember and even made a few humorous remarks. Helping them helped me.

It's funny; when others tried to play down the seriousness of the situation, I revolted.

"How dare they. What do they know," I would think. But when I did it, it was calming. Life is ironic sometimes.

While in the waiting room of the surgeon's office the following day, I had a reality check. There were patients with serious cancers and major surgeries waiting to be seen. We shared a few quick stories and mine seemed minor in comparison. I tried to put it all in perspective and was grateful for all the positive things that had happened this past week.

Dr. Preston was supportive and seemed to think it was a matter of some radiation treatments. My official diagnosis, he explained, was invasive ductal carcinoma grade 2. I didn't know what it all really meant, but I didn't say anything at the time.

"Frankly, I am surprised at the report," he said. "It didn't look like much when we removed it. It was so small and the margins were all clear so that means we got it all out. You just need an oncologist to set up your treatment plan. Do you know who you want?"

One good thing about working in healthcare is having the connections of your peers. Once I knew I needed an oncologist, I called my friend from the research council. She worked in the cancer center, and I trusted her judgment completely.

Many times, people would call me when they needed a cardiologist or a cardiac surgeon, and I had no problem giving my recommendation. Now it was my turn to ask.

"Dr. Burton," she said without hesitation. Dr. Burton it was.

When I said the name of the oncologist I had chosen, the surgeon hesitated.

"I have to forewarn you. He will be aggressive in his treatment."

"Aggressive treatment and cancer… I think that is a winning combination," I said with confidence.

"Okay," he said. "I will send your records to his office."

My hematoma was still painful but I left feeling good about my decision. As I headed back to work, I began to ponder the words… cancer… oncologist… aggressive; my confidence began to wither.

I then did what I always do when I begin to lose sight of a situation; I called my sister, and then I made a reservation to go to California. I wanted to see my boys.

Chapter 15
Complicating the Situation

At one time or another, we all have had that aggravating experience of trying to make an appointment. I called the cable company the other day and had to go through seven menus before I finally got to a human voice on the other end.

It is so frustrating to us who can actually understand the system, but think how difficult it must be for the elderly and for those who cannot maneuver through the prompts just to talk to a real person.

I remember my mom trying to make a simple doctor's appointment and finally calling me and asking if I would do it for her. If I had any recommendations for office personnel who answer the phones in a medical workplace, it is to not lose sight of the fact that the person on the other end is an individual who might be scared.

I tried to establish an appointment with the oncologist as soon as possible, but, in the end, I am not too proud to say I by-passed all those hassles and used my connections to be seen as soon as possible. I called my friend in the cancer center.

After a few moments of small talk, I finally said, "I took the recommendation you gave me for an oncologist, but I am having a hard time getting an appointment here in the cancer center to see him."

The physicians have their own offices where they see patients; but in addition, they come once a week to the hospital cancer centers to care for people as well. "I figure since I work here, I might as well try to see him on his scheduled day in this facility instead of driving across town."

"Of course," she responded eagerly. "Let me call you back."

A few minutes later, my phone rang. "You are scheduled this Friday at 10 a.m."

I have to admit I felt a little guilty about getting an appointment so soon in this manner, but relieved at the same time. A few weeks of radiation and it would all be over.

My sister offered to go with me, but I declined.

"I am just going to talk to him. I appreciate the offer, but I will be fine. I'll call you as soon as I get back."

I went down to the cancer center on D Level a little early Friday morning. I am always on time for appointments, but this day I was obviously more anxious that usual. The only time I had been on this level of the hospital was to use the conference room down there, so I didn't really know my way around.

I always saw the Cancer Center sign when I went to my meetings, but I didn't think much about it until now. I would notice patients moving in and out, but the thought of what a cancer patient experienced was not on my radar screen until I became one.

After signing in, I was told to go to the waiting room and someone would come to get me shortly. It is a strange feeling for a nurse to sit in a hospital waiting room. Usually we control the flow of patients but this day, I was the one being controlled.

Every magazine I picked up had a cancer theme to it, and, as I thumbed through them, I thought to myself, "This isn't about me. I only need some radiation. I don't really have cancer anymore, so to speak; just a small spot that they already cut out." Denial is a wonderful thing.

Just a minute or two later, someone came to get me. She was gracious and caring, and we chatted about work for a few minutes before beginning the registration. The questions involved a family history as well as the insurance information, and then we walked toward the back. I saw the radiation oncology sign to the right and the medical oncology one to the left.

"Dr Burton will see you in a minute, but we need to do a few things first. Can you sit in the scale please?"

It is extremely humbling to step up and sit down in a chair that is attached to a scale, while many of your peers are gathered around. One took my blood pressure and another my temperature, but all I cared about at this point was my weight.

I had just lost several pounds and my weight at home on my scale was finally acceptable to me, but to get weighed sitting in a chair out in the open with my back to the display screen was another story.

"139," the technician said out loud.

"Okay, let's just tell the entire hospital," I said grinning at him as I got up quickly.

We both laughed, but I was half serious. Weight is a very private matter to women, and I was no exception. After all the measurements were charted, I was taken back to the examination room.

"Take off everything from the waist up," the nurse explained, "and put on this gown. Dr. Burton will be in shortly. You look great, Judi."

"Thanks," I said in return.

As I waited, many of the staff nurses came in to see me. I knew several of them from the committees I had attended over the years, and they wanted to say hello and show their support.

As I tried to hold the gown closed enough as to not expose myself to my peers and yet be able to hug them at the same time, I thanked them for their help.

"What happened?"

"How did you find this?"

"You have the best doctor there is for breast cancer."

"I am sorry to hear about your diagnosis, but you are in good hands."

All the questions and comments made the time quickly pass by, but before I could explain that I didn't have breast cancer any more, the physician assistant came in to see me.

She sat and talked to me for a long time, explaining all the different procedures and plans of care for this type of cancer.

"I know Dr. Burton pretty well, and I think I know what he will want to do, but he will make those decisions with you, not me."

"The surgeon said maybe just radiation," I tried to explain again.

"We'll see," she said as she washed her hands and smiled warmly.

A quiet, unassuming man, I immediately liked him. I could tell he cared about his patients and wanted to do everything right for me. We talked about my biopsy surgery, my hematoma, the best and the worst scenarios that could happen from here forward, my expectations for just radiation, and his admitted aggressive treatment plans.

He explained things in simple terms; just because I was a nurse, did not mean that I knew anything about cancer language.

I had asked for a copy of my pathology report before I left for California, but I did not recognize any of the jargon. Jeff had given me a book that explained everything about breast cancer and the treatments in layman terms, so it really helped me to understand some of the terminology, but it wasn't my area of expertise.

I remembered when we had a new mother on our unit who had cardiac disease. They wanted her heart monitored, so after she delivered her baby, they brought her to us. We all were a little nervous about taking care of a mother and a baby.

"Give me a good old heart attack any day," I said jokingly to my manager. "I am more comfortable with that."

That is how I felt about the language they spoke down on D Level. A nurse is not a nurse is not a nurse; we all have our specialties and this was not mine. Plus, when a nurse is a patient, all rational thinking goes out the window anyway. We need things uncomplicated and straight-forward just like everyone else.

When I did patient care and would help patients to the bathroom, they would always be embarrassed by any exposure of themselves when we had to clean them up. We constantly tried to ease their fears and tell them that is why we were there, but it was apparent that they were humiliated.

I experienced that exact feeling when I had to have a breast exam on this day. I understand, just as my patients did, that physicians see many breasts and there was nothing special about mine...except that they were mine.

Dr. Burton and the staff were professional in every sense of the word, but having to expose myself to my peers was difficult. I was glad when I could get back into my own clothes and back to some control of my situation.

After I got dressed, we met again to talk. I realized then that this was going to be more than I anticipated.

Dr. Burton explained the difficult situation of my course of action. My tumor was very small as far as tumor sizes go, but right on the cusp of one way of thinking versus the other.

Usually, tumors this size or smaller are treated with only radiation, just as I had expected. But when the cancer area is just a millimeter larger, the plan included a lymph node biopsy.

"You are too young and too healthy not to be aggressive," he explained. "We discussed your case at tumor board last week and all but one physician agreed you should have a sentinel node biopsy just to be sure."

I was surprised to know my case was talked about at tumor board.

I only knew about these discussions because I would see all the food outside the classroom each week.

"What goes on in there?" I asked one day. "Who gets all that good food while they are meeting?"

"Tumor board," my friend replied. "They confer about each case, show the films, and discuss the proper course of action for each patient."

"Great," I thought to myself as we talked. "My breast was up on the screen in the classroom at my work place."

"Is this going to be another surgery?" I asked, already knowing the answer.

I went back upstairs to work and began the calls again. Everyone had the same opinion as we talked; "At least you will know and not have to worry whether you have cancer anywhere else."

"I am glad he isn't taking any chances."

And last but not least, my favorite quote, "It is better to be safe than sorry."

The encouragement was extremely nice and very much appreciated, but I just didn't want to have surgery again.

By now three weeks had past and I still had no resolution to this situation that started with a white dot on an x-ray. I remembered patients telling me how they had been cutting grass one day and having heart surgery the next, and how difficult it was to adjust to such a dramatic change so quickly. My process was long and tedious, and I wasn't sure which one was worse.

As I worked throughout the day, I told more and more of my co-workers the change in plans. Everyone supported the idea that it was better to do it all now and know that everything is okay.

On the drive home that evening, I tried to put it all in perspective and be grateful for the good healthcare and support that I had. I remembered Rob and his positive outlook; even when things looked bleak, he saw the glass half full and never complained.

"It beats the alternative," he would say jovially when the news wasn't so good. If he were here, that is exactly what he would say to me before he asked me if I wanted any ice cream. He was always trying to get me to eat ice cream with him. I smiled; He was my role model.

"I miss you, Rob," I said out loud.

Chapter 16
Macaroni and Cheese

My flight to California wasn't for a few weeks, so I decided to get my sentinel node biopsy before my trip.

"That way," I said in a text message to my sons, "We can celebrate in paradise."

Yes, at my age, I could actually use the texting feature on my phone! On one trip out to the west coast, Jeff and Adam told me to let them know when I landed. They lived close enough to the airport that, by the time I got off and got my luggage, they could be there to pick me up. As the attendant announced that we could use our phones, I typed in both of their phone numbers and proclaimed, "I'm here!"

Adam told me later they discussed on the way to the airport how surprised they were that I knew how to send a message to two people at the same time. "Hey. I am more than just a pretty face," I said laughing at their story.

I really did refer to their place of residence paradise. Being from the mid-west, I considered the weather in southern California heavenly. Not too hot or cold, a nice breeze, beautiful parks, great shopping and spectacular sightseeing.

Whenever I visited, I took long walks every morning, which was a welcomed change from the constant beating of the treadmill that I did every day at home.

In the evenings, we would all socialize together as a family as we sat out on the patio having a glass of wine. Oh, the good life. I was looking forward to getting this all behind me and heading out across the country to paradise.

The morning of the biopsy, I had to go back to the Breast Center before going to surgery. It seemed everything I had to do was more complicated than I had anticipated. The doctor explained that a sentinel lymph node biopsy included an injection of a radioactive blue colored dye into the skin right before the surgery. The sentinel nodes are the first few lymph nodes that drain fluid from the breast, so if the cancer cells had extended out past the breast ducts, these are the ones that would forewarn that the cancer cells had spread into the lymph system.

After the injection, the surgeon can then use a hand held probe that can identify which lymph nodes contained the radioactive substance, while the blue dye stained the first few nodes as well. After determining which ones are the sentinel nodes, the surgeon can then remove them for testing.

Sounded reasonable to me. I just wanted it over and done with.

It took longer than expected for the nuclear tech to bring the vials for injection. The radiologist, the technician, and I waited patiently for the materials to arrive, but in the meantime, I was half naked in front of my peers.

I knew there was no other choice. The skin had been prepped and if it was contaminated by any clothing, it would have to be repeated again.

We did the usual chitchat as they tried to make me feel as comfortable as possible, but I don't think there is anything that can take away that vulnerable feeling.

I remembered having discussions with my co-workers about some of the unusual body parts we had encountered as caretakers, and I wondered if my chest would be a topic of their conversation over lunch.

"Probably not," I thought chuckling to myself as I glanced down at my profile.

Finally the tech arrived with the vials, and the injection took only a minute or two to complete. I was given a card that said I had been exposed to a radioactive material and was told to keep it with me for 30 days. What a feeling to know you have been injected with a material that lights you up like a Christmas tree!

I jokingly asked if I would set off the security system when I went to the airport the following week, and was told to just be sure I had the card with me when I traveled.

While I was deciding whether I should be worried about this or not, the technician said, "Okay. We are finished. I will walk you over to the surgery center."

My left breast lymph nodes were now draining the identifying radioactive fluid, and my skin was a pretty shade of blue.

"We have to quit meeting like this," I told the registrar at the desk as I signed in while still wearing my patient gown.

"Do you have someone with you today?" she asked, concerned.

"Oh, my sister is coming a little later. Could you send her back when she arrives?" I asked.

"Of course, honey," she replied quickly.

I knew the routine so I headed back toward the same day surgery area. As I walked past all of the people in the waiting room, I had an instant memory flash of Rob and the heart transplant waiting room.

"I wish you were here with me, Rob" I thought. He always kept me grounded.

Checked in, IV started, gown on; I was familiar with the routine.

As the nurse came in to do all the paperwork again, she got called to another room. There was some commotion going on out in the hallway, and they needed her help.

My sister arrived, some of my co-workers stopped by, and I made a few calls, but no one ever came back into the room. I checked my watch; I was supposed to go to surgery in 15 minutes and the pre-op checklist had not even been started. I was getting a little anxious. Did they forget me?

A few minutes later, the nurse came to the doorway.

"Dr. Preston is still tied up in surgery. His first case is taking longer than expected, so your surgery will be delayed. This is a good time for me to go to lunch. If they call for you before I get back, one of my colleagues will finish up in here."

She smiled and waved at me as she walked away with her friend, discussing the macaroni and cheese that was on the menu that day.

I was stunned. "Lunch?" I thought to myself. How could she go to lunch when I wasn't anywhere near ready for surgery, and, didn't she know I was having a lymph node biopsy?? A biopsy for cancer, for God's sake! Let's see...... macaroni and cheese versus cancer......what is more important??!!

For a moment, I was furious. It felt like lunch had a higher priority than my cancer biopsy, and then it suddenly occurred to me....that issue with my dating story and the patient.

I recalled his behavior when he thought my love life took precedence over his physical condition and my surprise when Adam, a young boy, agreed with him. I now understood it! I not only recognized it, I was living it!

When I thought of it from a nursing perspective, it made perfect sense. The doctor was tied up and surgeries were delayed, so it was a great time for her to go to lunch. I had done it many times in my career.

But when you are the patient facing a health situation, any deviation from your state of affairs seems impersonal and demeaning. It was eye opening to me.

I tried to explain my revelation to Donna, but I realized she didn't fully grasp my situation because she wasn't in it.

"Of course she went to lunch. What did you think she should do?"

I couldn't verbalize the feeling. My mind knew that sometimes surgeries take longer than expected; that even nurses have to eat; that she did everything correctly by explaining what she was doing and who would be covering for her. I did the exact thing every day as a nurse. But as a patient, my heart and mind said, "What about me?"

As my mind raced with new ideas and thoughts, a voice bellowed from the doorway.

"I'm back! I'll find out how much longer it might be for you, and then we will complete your checklist."

My nurse had returned from lunch, and I was still fine. Things would be taken care of and all was well. I had to laugh at myself for the childish thinking I had resorted to for a few minutes but also realized how fundamental this need was in all of us.

When I was a family member, I acted as a family member; when I was a nurse, I thought like a nurse; and now as a patient, I was behaving like so many patients I had encountered throughout my professional life.

I recalled asking a patient one day how his night went.

"It was awful. I was awake most of the night because there was all this turmoil in the room next door. I could hear the nurses talking to the other guy and trying to fix his breathing problems. I think he eventually ended up going to the ICU but it was very late. I really didn't want to hear about anyone else's troubles; I have enough of my own."

At the time I remember thinking how selfish that was. After all, he was a patient too and the nurses were just taking care of an emergent situation. That was their job. He would expect the same treatment if it were him, wouldn't he?

Now, here I was, not really caring to hear about the hip replacement next door or wanting my nurse to go to lunch. I wanted them to concentrate only on me and my situation. It was like falling into survival mode.

This brought to mind the only other time I had been hospitalized. It was about a year after Rob had died, and I was having some physical symptoms. I had all the tests to rule out the bad stuff; EKG, blood tests, ultrasound, stress test. Everything was normal yet I was still dizzy and having recorded heart palpitations.

As the symptoms increased, I got more and more upset about the situation. I was having financial concerns in addition to the health condition I was experiencing, and I could not afford to get sick—both for myself and for the sake of the boys.

As time progressed, I started to cry; cry out of frustration, sadness, fear, and a whole litany of reasons I didn't even understand. And once I began to cry, I wasn't able to stop. I cried at work; I cried at home. There was no controlling the flood of emotions that were surfacing and my crying was spiraling out of control.

My doctor eventually suggested that it might be psychologically based and that I might need some professional help to manage the stress of widowhood, school, and single parenting. Taking medications was one thing, but when he suggested being hospitalized for a week or so, I cried even harder.

"You have been through hell and you just need a little rest," he said calmly. "You have not taken the time to grieve so your body is telling you through physical symptoms that it can't take any more. Take a few weeks and allow yourself to heal." I had no other answers, so I agreed.

Jeff happened to be home from college for a visit, so I went in and woke him up early that Sunday morning.

"I have to leave for a little while to go get better. Please help take care of your brother and I will be back soon."

My mom and step dad picked up Adam and Jeff and promised me they would be fine. I then called my sister. We drove to the hospital in silence except for my crying, and she said leaving me there was the hardest thing she ever had to do.

The two weeks that I spent in that place taught me firsthand about survival mode. I had no idea what to expect, but it wasn't what I discovered.

When faced with a medical situation that seemed frightening and out of control, I became self-centered and self-absorbed. The smallest inconvenience became a major catastrophe, and the most important thing at the time was to get things back to exactly the way they were before the admission. I spent my time complaining about small things because I was too scared to face the obvious one.

I took the medication and was discharged to home, but it wasn't until I was ready to see the whole picture that I actually was healed.

When a patient is in survival mode, the real issue is replaced with a smaller insignificant one so that there is a perception of control. The real problem is just too scary.

I was placing all of my fears about this surgery on my nurse going to lunch because I could do something about that. I had witnessed so many of my patients doing the same thing when faced with an illness, but I never thought I could fall into the same state of mind so easily.

I always knew that the temperature of the food or the frequency of bowel functions were not as important as they became to many hospitalized patients, but I never understood that deep rooted fear and lack of control over the illness was at the core of it all.

"Baptism by fire," I said out loud, describing my experience of being a patient first hand.

"I have your pre-op medications," the nurse said as she entered the room. "They are finally ready for you." It was now 2 p.m. and my surgery was originally scheduled for 11 a.m.

"Did the doctor get to eat lunch?" I asked worriedly as I watched her inject the clear liquid into my IV line. Hey, just because I understood the rationale of my behavior didn't mean I could change it. I first worried about my nurse going to lunch and now I was concerned about whether or not my doctor had enough time to take nourishment.

"See you later, alligator," I said as I glanced over at Donna and squeezed her hand.

"After while, crocodile," she answered as she kissed me on the forehead.

As I rolled into the OR and the narcotics were beginning to take effect, I noticed that my anesthesiologist was a former colleague of mine. We had worked together as staff nurses for about a year before he left to go back to anesthesia school.

"Hi, Mark," I said in a loud silly voice. I knew I was slurring my words but at this point, I didn't care. "You know my nurrrrr…." I started to tell him the story of my nursing instructor and knowing your anesthesiologist, but I couldn't finish my thought process. The drugs were kicking in, and I could barely slide over from the stretcher to the OR table.

As my eyes fluttered shut, my surgeon came in and smiled at me right before I drifted off into a dream state. My last image before finally going to sleep was seeing my nurse and my surgeon eating macaroni and cheese together in the cafeteria.

Chapter 17
The Final Diagnosis

"*D*o you want to go see Liz and the baby?" I asked Becky one afternoon as we were working on the schedule. Liz was one of our co-workers, and she had delivered a healthy baby boy the day before. We try not to interfere in people's personal lives, but when one of our peers has a baby, we all get excited.

"Sure,' she answered. "Let's call and see what time is good for her."

It had been a few days since my biopsy and I was waiting for the results. I had called the office but was told they were not available yet.

"I will call you as soon as we get them," the office nurse told me. Between my many visits to the physician and our common bond of working in the same institution, we had come to know each other on a first name basis.

After the biopsy, my sister met with the surgeon, and he acknowledged that the sentinel nodes were clearly marked and easy to find.

"They looked pretty normal," she was told and passed on that information to me. I was so happy. Finally, this ordeal was almost over and I could move on.

I had returned to school to get my Master's degree and I really needed to get back on track. And, I was looking forward to a trip out to the sunny west coast during this dreary winter season.

The baby was adorable, and Liz was beaming with pride. I was sitting in the rocking chair holding the newborn and we were all having a good time. My phone rang, and, as I handed the baby to Becky, I heard a familiar voice on the other end.

"Mrs. Schofield?"

"Yes," I responded quickly, knowing it was the nurse from the surgeon's office.

"We don't normally do this, but I knew you were anxious to get your results and I told you I would call as soon as they were in. I just came into the office and they are coming across the fax machine as we speak, so if you hold on for a minute, we will know them at the same time."

"Thank you so much. I really appreciate it," I whispered softly. I knew she was going out on a limb for me and I wanted her to know how grateful I was.

As I stepped out of the room and into the hallway for privacy, she began; "let's see, first sentinel node negative." I held my breath and felt my temples pulsating. "Second node negative." I smiled slightly, afraid to express my emotions just yet.

"Third node...wait a minute...what? Wait....oh, hell Judi. It says it is positive. One damn millimeter positive. I am so sorry. Maybe I should have waited...I don't know."

The apprehension in her voice was obvious, but I could not reassure her right now. Holding on to the handrail to keep from sliding down the wall, I vaguely remember finishing our conversation.

After we hung up, I took a few minutes to pull myself together and went back in to say goodbye to Liz. No need to spoil her happy day.

As Becky and I walked down the hallway to go back to the unit, I said calmly and mechanically, "my lymph node biopsy was positive. I think I just bought myself chemotherapy."

I looked straight ahead as we walked; I could not make eye contact with her right now. I knew if I did I would lose all control, and that wouldn't be fair to all those happy families on the mother baby unit. The circle of life wasn't so important to me at this minute. Here I was surrounded by all this new life while mine had just been shattered. The vulnerability was just too much too take.

As a nurse, I had been present many times when a patient received a medical diagnosis. My heart always went out to them, and I would try to support them in any way that I could. After all, I had also been there when Rob had his heart transplant, and I thought I knew what it was like to experience this trauma first hand.

But when you are the one on the receiving end of a life-threatening illness, words cannot describe the effect on your being. I thought I had lived through and understood most medical situations and the outcomes from them, but until you are the one in the bed, that is impossible to think, know, or feel.

It is like having the rug pulled out from beneath you and your footing on this earth lost. What you always knew as real is now confused and murky. Family and friends can surround and support you, but in the end, you are still alone with a cloud of uncertainty following you like a vague shadow at dusk.

It really is just a matter of perception; after all, no disease appears overnight. My oncologist told me that I probably had this cancer for a few years but that it took this long to find and diagnosis it.

I thought of my cardiac patients and knew that those problems took years to accumulate, but those people had lived a normal life until the onset of chest pain.

When we perceive that we are healthy, we live that way until we know otherwise. I now knew otherwise, and it changed my entire perception.

Becky and I traveled the nine floors down in silence, and I was grateful for her understanding that I couldn't talk about it right now.

The trip back to work seemed endless, and I was thankful when I finally made it back to my desk despite my wobbly knees.

I took a deep breath and then slowly picked up the phone to make the calls, first to my sister, then to my boys, and finally to my oncologist for an appointment. I was now back in list mode and I needed to know what was next. I had been knocked at the knees but I wasn't down yet.

At least that is what I said when I told people about my biopsy.

"It was only a millimeter," I said to Jeff and Adam. "How much harm can a little millimeter cause?" It made them feel better to think I had not lost my sense of humor.

By the end of the day, I had a PET scan scheduled for Friday, my sister said she would be with me every step of the way, and my director offered all the help and support from my work family that I needed. It seemed all things were falling into place except for me and my head.

Up to this point, I had not been able to cry, but I was so very sad. Not so much for me but for all of my choices and regrets.

It is human nature for us to go along and live day by day until something comes along to derail us. When I heard that I had cancer in my lymph node, I had a life review flashback.

Over the course of the next few days, I remembered things like being aggravated with Jeff over a silly little lunch box and making Adam feel bad over a girlfriend incident. I saw vivid images of their little faces, and my heart ached; why did those things seem so important at the time and now on a scale of significance, didn't matter at all.

I thought of all my patients who were so unreasonable and I found myself now understanding the anxiety and the irrational behavior they demonstrated when they were faced with a medical situation that had knocked them off their course. Dear God, give me a second chance.

Dr. Burton and I had a long talk. I can still hear his answer when I asked if one millimeter was worth going through the recommended treatment.

"One millimeter or a hundred millimeters; it doesn't matter," he said emphatically while looking over the top of his glasses.

"It is in your lymph node. You don't want to take the chance of one cell getting out there and spreading. Let's just attack it head on now and be sure."

I had no reason to doubt him; he was a good man and a highly respected physician in his field. I knew everything he said made sense, but it sounded so very scary.

Thoughts rushed through my head: would I miss work? Could I take care of myself? How sick would I be? And my hair…oh lord, would I lose my hair?

The answers to my questions and a lot more information was given to me that day. My sister asked if I wanted her to go with me, but I declined, thinking it was just an appointment to talk. In hindsight, I wished I had taken her up on her offer.

There was so much to take in and absorb that I regretted not having someone with me to help with information overload. It all worked out, though, and in the end, I left with a plan.

I was going with the traditional "big guns" treatment as my friend who worked in the cancer center called it. Four treatments of Adriamycin and Cytoxan, better known as AC, and then four of Taxol followed by six weeks of radiation. The treatments were to be given IV every other week, and the radiation schedule would be five days a week.

I would not need more surgery since the original breast biopsy had clear margins, meaning they had "gotten it all," unless, of course, I opted for a mastectomy.

We then talked at length about mastectomy vs. lumpectomy. The statistics demonstrated that if I followed this plan with my lumpectomy, chances of re-occurrence were single digit. I had a little time to make that decision because the chemotherapy treatment would be first no matter what the choice, but it was just another thing to worry about.

In order for all this to get started, I needed a port placement. This is something placed under the skin for IV use and for lab draws. It would prevent me from having to be stuck with a new IV each treatment; I was told the port was a cancer patient's best friend.

I also needed a PET scan to see if the cancer had spread anywhere else in my body and a cardiac echo to be sure my heart was in good shape. Some of the chemo drugs were toxic to the heart so it is vital to be sure that the heart was healthy beforehand. All this and, I wanted to take my trip to California.

I was told I should not travel during the treatment phase because of the risk of infection, and I wanted to see my boys before I began this process.

So much to do and I wanted to get started because I wanted this to be over as soon as possible.

My port got placed, my echo was normal, my PET scan was completed, and my trip was coming up. I really wanted the results of the scan before I left so I could go to California with all my information. I wanted to enjoy being with my sons fully and completely.

After several calls with no success, I called my friend again.

"Can you see if they have my results?" I humbly asked.

A few hours later, the nurse from the office called me.

"This is not our normal practice. Dr. Burton always gives test results to his patients and he is not available today. I understand you are going to see your children so he has given me permission to share it with you."

"I appreciate it," is all I could think to say, a little embarrassed that she knew I had called my friend.

"Well, there were no signs of cancer anywhere else, but there were a few hot spots in the left breast. These are probably from the surgeries that you recently had. They show up as inflamed areas and can give a false positive." Taken back again by the results, I stumbled over a few questions.

"How do I know that for sure? What if it is more cancer? Does my treatment plan change?"

"You will have to talk to the doctor about those things, but the plan will remain the same. Chemotherapy is always the first treatment. You can talk to him about the rest of your concerns when you return."

Stunned again, I wasn't sure what to do. Was it good news? Bad news?

I remembered times when patients were given results while in the hospital. Knowing they were upset, I would try to get them to talk to me about their feelings. Most of their concerns were how they received the information and what to do with it when the doctor left.

I was in that position now and I wondered if I had given enough of my time and attention to their needs. Knowing what I knew now, "I can only hope," I said to myself.

I went home and packed. Ironically, I didn't call anyone that night, and the next day, I got up and headed over to the airport. "Hot spots," I kept repeating in my head. I had to sort it all out.

While waiting to board, I called Donna and bounced it all off of her. We talked so long, I almost missed my flight.

During the long trip across the country, I reflected over the last few months. My first mammogram had been taken in December and here it was, the end of February, and I still had no resolution. So many ups and downs, decisions, choices, regrets, memories.

I thought of Shay and the frustration she must have felt trying to get someone to listen, and my heart ached for her and her family.

My thoughts were interrupted by the attendant's announcement to put away all electronic devices. We landed without incident, and I headed to the baggage claim to find my luggage.

As I walked outside to wait for my ride, I saw the palm trees swaying in the warm evening breeze. Searching the busy parking area, I spotted the car and saw Jeff and Adam both smiling and waving at me. A surge of fear, relief, anger, sadness, and a multitude of other emotions came crashing down like the Pacific Ocean at high tide.

As I ran toward the car, I began to cry. Cry and cry and cry. Finally, all of the pent up feelings and sensations were released and all it took was two beautiful faces and a warm California breeze.

In between the sobs, I told them all the stories. The ups and downs stories; the good and bad stories. The story of Shay. I realized how much I missed them being with me through all this, and I had two months of catching up to do. We talked and laughed and went out for a beer first and then ice cream and they helped me put it all into perspective.

That night I slept better than I had in months and went out for my walk the next morning. It felt so good to finally cry, but mostly it felt good to see my boys.

My last night there, we went out to dinner and I told them about the lunch box and the girl friend regrets. I apologized for those and all the others things I had done wrong over the years, and they both laughed and said they didn't even remember it. They made light of it all, and I thought maybe they were just trying to make me feel better. Either way, it worked. I got on the plane the next day with a renewed spirit and a light heart.

As we flew over the beautiful snowcapped mountains, I made a mental promise to myself to go back and do whatever was best for me and my health. I wanted to live to see my grandchildren born and take what I had learned as a patient back to my nursing career.

"Thank you, Rob, for those two great guys," I murmured as a prayer.

Chapter 18
A Dose of Reality

My first treatment was March 16th. I asked for Friday afternoon appointments because I was determined to keep my life as normal as possible, and staying on a schedule helped me to do that. This way, I could have the weekend to recover while trying to maintain an ordinary work life. Donna came to my office a little early and brought me a present.

"I am going to bring you a gift each time you have a treatment," she said smiling as she handed me a bag. A cute yellow sign that said "Gardening: there's magic in the dirt." I hugged her tightly.

"I hope I can get out in my yard this spring," I said hesitantly as I turned and shuffled some papers on my desk. Her gift brought tears to my eyes.

I loved the spring and summer months, and working in the yard was therapy for me.

"It's only four months," she said firmly.

"Easy for you to say," I thought to myself. "That takes me through July."

She glanced up at the clock.

"It is time to go," my sister said softly.

Being a nurse and a patient at the same time is torturous. As a nurse, we see every situation, reaction, and side effect known to humankind. We share our stories with each other because no one outside of the medical world would understand the sights and situations we witness.

Then when we have to slip out of work and into the patient mode, those memories come to the forefront. That was what was happening to me on the walk down the hall toward the elevator.

I was worried about having a drug reaction to all the new chemicals I was having injected into my body, and I wanted to talk to someone who understood my concern.

"I forgot one thing," I said to Donna as I stopped and handed her my purse. "I will be right back."

I briskly headed toward a few of my co-workers I saw standing in the corridor.

"I am going down to the Cancer Center to get my first chemo treatment. If the code light goes off down there over the next couple of hours, I want you to come down as quickly as you can. I want you there if something happens."

I think they normally would have laughed and thought I was kidding, but my body language and the urgency in my voice made them think otherwise.

"I promise," they said as we did a group hug. Okay. I felt better.

After signing in, I went through the ritual that would become second nature to me. Sitting in that horrible chair scale where everyone can see your weight, vital signs, the walk back to one of the patient rooms, blood work drawn from my port, and all the friendly greetings and smiles from the staff was always the beginning of my treatment schedule.

There was a recliner in each room where the patient could sit and relax during the visit and chairs for any other visitors. Family and friends were welcome and the nurses would come to know them as well as the patients. Looking around the room, I wondered how many others came before me and sat in this very chair. Were they healthy? Did it work?

I thought of all those patients who blazed the trail for the rest of us; who didn't have all the technical wonders and drugs available to them and often died of the side effects of the treatment.

"Are you ready to get started?" my nurse asked me as I was startled back to reality.

"Let's do it," I said with a knot as big as a fist planted firmly in my chest.

Tears began to well up in Donna's eyes as she watched the nurse begin. The drugs that I was going to receive were very toxic so the nurse had to wear protective gear while working with them.

"Here she was," she told me that evening, "wearing a mask and big thick gloves while scrubbing the skin over your port and putting the medication into your vein. It broke my heart to just sit and do nothing. I felt helpless." I remembered that feeling with Rob and I nodded my head in empathy.

The first things to be injected into my port were all the pre-treatment meds to prevent a reaction: Benadryl, decadron, ativan. Then I was given Emend by mouth for the post treatment nausea.

"Poison," I thought to myself as I closed my eyes. "This stuff is poison. I hate every minute of this," I said as the nurse brought in the first bag of IV fluids. "One damn millimeter," I thought to myself.

As she swabbed the skin again, she explained that the next step was going to be the Adriamycin or "red devil" as they called it, followed by the Cytoxan. This would be the process for my first four treatments every other week.

"The end of April," I calculated in my head. "Then the Taxol."

I watched as the bag was hung and threaded through the IV pump. We had just switched over to the new pumps, and the nursing staff was a little slow in getting used to them. Everyone had attended an in-service on the new system, but until you actually used them a few times, it took longer than usual.

"I don't like these new pumps," the nurse said as she pushed some buttons. "I am going to get Cindy to help me. She is good at this."

My heart skipped a beat as I recalled that just two days earlier, I had done the same thing. A pump was beeping, and I went in to fix it. Since I wasn't out on the unit every day, I did not remember how to clear the error so I went for help.

"I'll be right back," I said smiling at the patient. "These are new, and I need some help with this process."

I distinctly recalled the look of worry on his face when we returned.

"You think he'd be glad I went for help," I remember saying to the nurse who fixed it quickly for me. Now I was looking at Donna in panic.

Cindy came in, and in no time the red liquid was dripping into the chamber and slowly making its way down the tubing. I noticed a small air bubble in the midst of the liquid and followed it all the way to my port. Drip. Drip.

The closer it got to the end of the hose-like tubing, the more anxious I became.

I had to physically grip the arms of the chair to keep from jumping up and screaming, "There's an air bubble going into my body!" All my rational thinking as a nurse reminded me that I knew it was fine; that a small air bubble was commonplace and no cause of any harm. I had manipulated IV tubing hundreds of times in the past and explained the safety of the presence of a small air pocket, but as a patient, I couldn't process that information.

I was at the mercy of someone placing in me poison that could cause a life threatening reaction through a pump that no one knew how to use, and I just couldn't handle it all. Thank goodness for the quick action of the Ativan.

Just as I was about to make a fool of myself, I became so sleepy, I couldn't get the words out.

"Say goodnight to Judi," the nurse said to Donna as my eyes slowly closed. I tried to talk, but I was just too tired.

"An afternoon of fun and games," I said to my sister sarcastically as we walked to the car. I was still feeling a little loopy from the Ativan, but other than that, I was okay.

I thought back to my conversation with my friends about the code light vigil, and I had to smile.

"No reaction," I said calling the unit from my cell phone. They all wished me well and told me how proud they were of me. Little did they know how close I came to being one of those out of control patients we talked about at work.

First-hand experience at being a patient was enlightening to me. When we find ourselves in a compromised position, many of us bargain with God, and I was no exception.

"I will approach my work with a better understanding and appreciation if I survive this disease," I said silently as I glanced up at the dark clouds scattered throughout the late afternoon sky.

Over the next sixteen weeks, Donna and I developed a ritual that would become such a comfort to me. After all eight treatments, we went out to dinner and then back to my house. I would curl up on the couch and doze off and on while she sat on the loveseat and worked on her computer.

We always called our sister in Tacoma, Washington to give her an update of each treatment and the side effects I had encountered that week, and then try to stay awake to watch TV.

She spent the night with me because I had to return Saturday morning after each treatment for a shot of Nulasta. This was an injection that stimulated the production of white blood cells which are destroyed by the chemotherapy.

In the past, patient's blood counts would get so low that they would have to be hospitalized but with the discovery of drugs like this, that was now preventable. Everything comes with a price, though. Besides the high financial cost, the side effects were painful. About 24 hours after the injection, my bones would begin to ache severely.

Many times I had to take pain medication and go to bed to escape my throbbing arms and legs, but after a few days, the soreness subsided. Some weeks the side effects were worse than others, but each time, we did the same thing.

I received a new gift with all eight treatments, and the nursing staff was just as excited as I was to see what was in the bag.

On the Friday of my second treatment, Jeff came home to go to the Cancer Center with me. It was such a pleasant surprise to see him and have him with me during this time. I liked that the drugs made me fall asleep, but I hated that Donna would then sit there by herself, so knowing she had Jeff to talk to made me feel better as well.

At the same time, a nurse friend of mine called and offered to do Raiki for me. I knew she had done healing touch work for some of her patients in the past, but now she said she would be happy to come to the Cancer Center to provide it for me.

"Sure," I said, thanking her on the phone.

"I'm going to go get my poison," I said to Becky as we left the unit. Donna, Jeff, Danielle, and I all headed toward the elevator.

"Can I talk to you a minute?" Danielle said to me as we completed the registration and were seated in a room big enough to accommodate all of us.

"Of course," I answered quickly. We had known each other many years and I respected her as a nurse and a friend.

"I wish you wouldn't call the medications poison," she began. "These drugs are a blessing to you. They are giving you new life."

She went on to remind me about having a positive attitude and the effect it has on the healing process.

"You know, all the stuff we tell our patients," she said as she gently patted my hand.

We discussed the power of visualization and being in synch with our bodies.

"Attitude is everything," she reminded me.

Her frankness with me brought me back to a place of comfort and peace. A position of letting go of the fear and anxiety and just being in the moment.

As the chemo bag was hung, I closed my eyes and pictured it flowing through my body like a white light overtaking all the dark cancer cells. I didn't worry about the pump or the air bubble, but instead visualized pac man-like molecules swallowing anything in their way to clear a path for the healing fluid to flow.

I felt her soft hands upon my shoulders and imagined her energy combining with mine to remove all the anger and fear and anxiety.

On that day, I made peace with my cancer and my chemotherapy. I called it a blessing, not a poison.

Combining my experience as a family member, a nurse, and now a patient, I could trust that all these things came together for something good.

My side effects were no different than the first treatment; nausea, bone pain, fatigue. The difference was in my reaction to them. Instead of fighting it, I took my meds, ate well and drank green tea, and just tried to live in the midst of acceptance.

"This too shall pass," was my motto any time I would get discouraged.

I napped when I needed to but always got up and went to work. I continued to attend my nursing classes and soaked up all the love and friendship that was extended to me. Staying active was very important to me so I tried to keep up an exercise routine at a level I could handle.

I not only received the eight gifts of love from my sister but also the gifts of family, friends, and gratitude for modern medical science.

Many take life for granted until a health diagnosis brings with it the fear of the unknown and the challenges of the human spirit. If we understood the reaction of those in each medical situation and communicated with each other like Danielle did with me that day, we could bring all aspects of healthcare to a community level. And when two or more gather together for the same cause, anything is possible.

Chapter 19
Baldness and Balance

"*O*kay, let's do it," I said to Jeff and Donna on one Sunday afternoon as we were finishing our lunch at the local chili parlor. It was the Sunday after my second treatment and the nausea was pretty bad. It sounded strange, but I needed something like spaghetti to settle my stomach.

After a few bites though, I decided it wasn't such a good choice so I just sipped on my drink while I waited for them to finish their meal.

"Ironic,' I thought to myself. It is April 1st. April Fool's Day.

During my initial visit to the oncologist, I was told my hair would start to fall out after or about the time of the second treatment. We all believe at one time or another that the rules don't apply to us, and I was no exception. Somewhere in the reservoir of my mind, I thought maybe, just maybe, mine would be different. But today, reality had met me head on—literally—and a decision to take control of the situation was made.

Ever since the second treatment on Friday, my hair had begun to come out by the handfuls. Pieces of hair scattered throughout my bed and a thin layer on the shower floor that morning were hard core evidence of the inevitable. I was losing my hair.

As we sat there, I told Jeff and Donna that I didn't want to find hair all over my house.

"Not only is it messy but it is degrading to just sit and wait for it to happen. It is not going to come out on its terms, it is coming out on mine," I said with wavering conviction.

"We could shave it off," Jeff responded quickly, and Donna looked at me to see my reaction.

It was a warm windy day that April 1st. As the three of us set out toward the back yard, we started with a little ceremony by taking some pictures and trying to find a sense of humor in this very personal situation.

Jeff brought out a chair from the kitchen and pulled an electric shaver from his luggage.

"I brought it just in case," he said smiling warmly. "I wanted to be here to help you through this."

As I sat in the chair, I rubbed my bare feet in the moist grass as a diversion to keep from crying. I suddenly remembered a time many years ago when I went to the beauty shop and was convinced that I would look good with an extremely short hair do. When I came home, my mom screamed, "What have you done to yourself? Where is your beautiful hair?"

It was extremely traumatic then but it quickly grew back and the incident eventually forgotten until now.

"My beautiful hair," I thought to myself as I held back the tears.

The motor hummed and I began to see hair flying all over the yard. The wind was furious that day, almost as if it was reacting to the emotions I felt inside.

"Good thing you haven't committed a crime," my sister said patting my shoulder. "Your DNA is blowing all over the city."

In just a few minutes, it was over. I rubbed my hand over my head and remembered the same sensation when I swept my hand over Adam's head each summer when he got his "buzzed" baseball haircut.

They brought me a mirror and I stared at the image. Surprisingly, it wasn't so bad. Jeff had left a small half inch layer of hair and it was very even and stylish.

"You have a perfectly shaped head," he said walking from back to front and evaluating the situation. He was so supportive.

The whole body image concern had come to light recently. When I was in nursing school, we would have a nursing diagnosis for each patient. Many times it was, "Alteration in body image related to..." whatever might be the patient's issue.

We witnessed this many times on our unit because of the nature of the surgical focus we had. Chest, arm, and leg incisions; tube and wire scars; multiple IV sticks and bruises. I understood the risk vs. necessity of it all, but I could see how it affected the patient's image of themselves.

As I looked in the mirror after my shower that night, I completely and fully understood it. My face looked foreign to me without my hair.

"G.I. Jane," I said out loud to myself.

"You could only wish you looked as good as Demi Moore did in that movie," I then thought humorously. I knew I would soon lose my eye brows and lashes which would be even more dramatic.

Looking down at my breast, I saw all the scars and depressions from the surgeries and the lump from the port. They may be only small disfigurements, but it was a completely different body than the one I had inhabited all these years. Despite all its flaws, it had carried me well.

Whether I was packed down with my "invisible suitcase" on my back or laughing hysterically with my friends, this body had carried me through it all. It held me upright at the head of Rob's casket and supported me through those long 12 hour shifts.

I missed it and I wanted it back just like the way it used to be. Like a comfortable pair of jeans; like my favorite wore-torn bathing suit or my warm and fuzzy robe; like Rob and the Pillsbury Doughboy. I got dressed and cried myself to sleep.

By May, I had completed the AC chemo and was now moving on to Taxol. One of the downsides to our healthcare system is the regulations set by insurance companies.

When I first started chemo, I had a prescription for an anti-nausea medication. Because it is expensive, my insurance required a special approval of it before it would cover any of the cost.

By the time I was discharged from the cancer center after my first treatment and went to the pharmacy with prescriptions in hand, the insurance company was closed. The pharmacist could not call for approval until Monday and I could not afford the high cost of filling the entire amount, so I had to compromise.

I remember standing over that counter feeling sick begging them to help me. I could not make it through the weekend without it; the nausea was overwhelming, so I ended up paying the full price of $200.00 for a few tablets to make it to Monday.

I had to ration them over Saturday and Sunday until the approval came and I could get the rest of the tablets. It is stressful enough to be sick without having to worry about how to afford needed medications.

Patients often told me they didn't take their meds because they were not able to pay for them, and there I was on a Friday night at the pharmacy living the same experience.

The Taxol treatments fit the same criteria. There were severe side effects to the approved version of the drug but because of the cost of the newer form, the approved one had to be tried first. The newer version could only be used if the side effects were bad enough to warrant its use.

After my first treatment, I had lost four toe nails and had a terrible neuropathy in my feet that is still present today. The side effects were sufficient to get the approval of the newer form called Abraxane, and my treatment plan was changed.

It is just a shame that patients have to experience situations such as this because of cost and insurance coverage, but that is the reality of our healthcare system.

Jeff made it home for three of my chemo treatments and Adam was able to make it for one. It was so nice to have them with me, and I knew it was difficult to get here all the way from California because of school schedules and travel time.

Having my loved ones there to support me helped to cope with the emotional aspect of my illness. Donna was always there with us and we spent our Friday nights together.

On the eighth and final treatment, we had a family celebration. Jeff brought me flowers and Donna had non-alcoholic grape juice ready to toast the completion of chemotherapy. We made calls to Jo and Adam to include all of our family in the celebration. One process down and one to go.

The next phase was radiation. It had been another one of those tough decisions. I contemplated having a mastectomy because of the fear of the return of the cancer, but after talking with my oncologist, I decided to do the radiation and not the surgery.

It is a very personal decision, and each individual needs to examine it from her own perspective and viewpoint. I knew if I had radiation and then needed a mastectomy later on, I could not have reconstructive surgery.

After weighing all the pros and cons, I made my decision but it was a difficult choice to make.

By now it was the beginning of July. I was completely bald and wearing a terrific wig that I had found on my trip to California. I only wore it to work or a social event, and the other times I just tied a scarf around my head.

I continued to go to cardiac rehab in the mornings to work out. For the last few years, I had done this, and I wanted to keep my life as routine as possible, Sometimes I only had enough energy to walk slowly on the treadmill, but at least I was moving. The social aspect was important to me as well.

My radiation oncologist was a nice man who was warm and friendly. After my chemo was completed, Dr. Burton asked who I wanted to manage my radiation treatments. Since I had no knowledge of any of these specialists, I asked for his opinion.

"To whom would you send your wife if she needed radiation?" A week later, I was sitting in the waiting room of the recommended physician.

He explained the process and all the side effects while I took it all in and nodded in understanding. By now, I was really trying to live as Danielle had said and "just accept what is; don't fight it but embrace it."

"When do we start?" I asked.

Before beginning any radiation treatments, the area has to be marked and a treatment plan designed. This is a precise procedure where a special x-ray machine is used to mark the exact place where the radiation will be directed. It is called simulation, and it is extremely important that it be accurate.

I was in the simulation room on a hard table with my arms above my head. My chest was exposed, and the technician was apologizing profusely. There were computer issues and if I moved, I would have to start over when it was fixed.

"I am so very sorry," she said standing next to me looking down at my face.

"It's okay," I said. It would do no good to get upset.

After an hour and a half of every attempt they could make, we finally had to quit.

"We just can't get it right, and I want it to be exact for you," the doctor said as he entered the room. "We will have to try again when the computer is fixed."

I tried to lower my arms in order to get up, but the pain was excruciating. They had been raised so long that it took two people to move them ever so slowly from its upright position to eventually down by my sides. My tolerance was waning but I smiled when I could finally get back to an upright position.

The following week, the simulation was ultimately completed but it was a grueling course of action.

"Be grateful for the treatment," I had to remember.

When I was finally ready to start the radiation treatments, I had marks all over my breast. There were clear plastic dressings covering them so they would not wash off, and I had a cream to use to help reduce the burns. Although it is such a precise method of treatment, it seemed so archaic in the administration of it.

Half way through my treatments, I met a woman who was also getting radiation. She was still very angry about her diagnosis and talked about her simulation experience.

"I felt like a cow being branded," she told me. "I hate all this."

"It's all a matter of perception," I tried to explain to her. "Just concentrate on being grateful."

It reminded me of patients that I had cared for as a nurse. They would get so angry over the smallest detail and I never understood why. Now as a patient, I know it is a complicated human reaction to lack of control over a perceived interpersonal situation.

The term "patient" comes from the Latin word "patiens" meaning "one who endures," Or "one who suffers." It is also a form of the word "patience." I now knew what it was like to experience that endurance, that suffering, that patience first hand.

Compared to the time it took to receive chemotherapy, radiation was much quicker. I went five days a week for six weeks, and it took longer to change clothes and sign in than it did for the treatment.

As I sat in the waiting room, I met so many people who struggled with facing their health crisis. Some of them had to take two or three buses back and forth just to get to their treatments, and others had no health insurance to cover the high costs.

One of the ladies had to be admitted to the hospital due to the side effects of her treatment and I thought about some of the patients I had admitted from the Cancer Center. I usually didn't think much about what they had been through before they got to me.

I was so concerned about treating their illness and getting them back to normal that I sometimes forgot about all the history they brought with them; their "invisible medical baggage" so to speak.

My son has a video game that tests the balance competency of the participants. As the virtual person walks out on a tightrope, the player has to not only keep him upright but also has to avoid the high winds and soaring pieces of debris that are trying to knock him down.

The stress of being a patient is like walking that tightrope in real life. And when things start flying in around them and it seems like the fall is unavoidable, gathering together as a safety net for each other is not just the right thing to do, it's the only thing to do.

Part Four:
Coming Full Circle

"Until he extends his circle of compassion to include all living things, man himself will not find peace."

— Albert Schweitzer

Chapter 20

Adam

The day was hectic as usual. As a manager of a busy cardiac unit, there were meetings and schedules and a million other things that filled the daylight hours. I looked out the window and saw that dusk had already settled in for the night. As I vowed to try to go home earlier in the future, the phone rang.

"Mom," I heard Adam's voice.

"Hi honey," I said smiling into the mouthpiece and sitting back down into my chair. "What's up?" I always enjoyed calls from my boys.

"It's time for my echocardiogram, and I don't have a cardiologist out here. My primary care doctor wants all the records from the cardiologist before she will refill my prescription. Can you help me figure it all out?"

I remember watching the movie "The March of the Penguins," and witnessing the unbearable conditions that the penguins endured. They suffered through the horrific elements of snow and blizzard-like conditions to ensure the safety of their eggs until they hatched.

I cried as they huddled together in unison, holding the eggs up on their feet to keep them from freezing on the ice, all for the safety and well-being of their offspring. That is how I felt about my boys.

I would do anything to help them but especially if it pertained to their health. I've always said that when I face my God at the end of my life and have to account for what I have done and not done, I will have my "ace in the hole."

When called upon to give an inventory of my life, my answer will be followed by, "But what about my boys, Lord; what about my boys? They are such fine young men."

My heart skipped a beat as I again flipped from being a manager to thinking like a nurse and then back to that frantic family member mode. Since Adam's diagnosis, I had to carefully balance the nurse and family member role in order to keep both in perspective, and I knew I would do him no good by reacting like I did in the past.

Hopefully I had learned a valuable lesson in medical humanity by experiencing all three sides of the hospital bed and remembering what it was like to be in each situation.

"Okay," I answered. "I'll do whatever I can to help you. Tell me the details."

After Rob's death, it was suggested that Adam have an echocardiogram because of the strong family history.

"This way, we will have something to compare it to when he grows up, and we can monitor him throughout his life to be sure it doesn't change. It is just a precaution." It was a reasonable suggestion so, at age seven, Adam had his first test.

The results were normal except for a very small deviation in one area.

"If I didn't know about his dad's disease, I would consider it completely normal," the doctor explained, "But since the family element is there, let's just repeat the echo annually." So that's what we did.

Every year, we would go to Children's Hospital for an echocardiogram and an exam by a cardiologist and every year, it was the same. Year after year, nothing changed. Until that year.

I had come home from work one evening and there was a voice mail from our primary care physician.

"Give me a call, Judi," was his only message. I had no idea why he would call me at home, but bright and early the next morning, I saw him in the hallway.

"Adam's test was a little abnormal," he said hesitantly after I questioned him about the vague phone call.

"How abnormal? What is his ejection fraction?" I asked frantically. This was a number that Rob and I had lived with and worried about throughout his entire illness. It is a measurement of the ability of the heart to pump blood effectively and could be the signal that something isn't right.

"I just want him to see a cardiologist to be on the safe side," he explained as we walked and talked simultaneously. "Call Dr. Clems and have him review it."

I could tell he was uncomfortable telling me any facts at the time and wanted a specialist to be involved in Adam's care. I appreciated his concern but I really wanted and needed some answers.

Before I had time to think, I saw Dr. Clems getting off the elevator. Literally running down the hall, I blurted out, "I need your help." We moved to a quiet corner of the unit and I explained what little I knew about the situation.

"I will go down and look at his films personally," he said trying to comfort me.

I was able to squeak out a weak "thank you," as I watched him walk toward the stairwell.

The next hour seemed like forever but eventually he came back to my office and stood in the doorway.

"His ejection fraction on his echo last week was 35%."

My heart sank. A normal result is anywhere between 55 to 70 percent. I wanted to scream and cry and display all the reactions we have when we hear bad news, especially anything pertaining to our children.

I tried to remember how I felt when I heard about Rob's heart disease, and my reaction as a patient to my cancer diagnosis and surgery, and lastly, how it felt to be a nurse witnessing other patients in these similar positions.

"You've come full circle, Judi. Take what you have learned from all these situations and be a help to Adam, not a hindrance," I thought to myself.

"What do we do now?" I asked calmly.

"Call my office and schedule an appointment for this week," he answered as he bent over and hugged me lightly. "It will be okay."

I sat in silence for a long time. "This just cannot be," I said to no one in the room. "I thought I was done."

I remembered thinking after Rob's death that I was immune to any other disaster or negative situation. Like an expiration date on tragedy. It had been a false sense of protection that took over and I thought, "Okay, I've had mine. At least it is someone else's turn now."

I believe it is a survival tactic that our minds use to make it through a traumatic event. When I was diagnosed with cancer, I knew in reality that we were all equally vulnerable and eventually accepted that the only thing I could control was my reaction to it. But this was testing every ounce of my inner strength.

Within a few days, Adam went to the cardiologist and had a battery of tests and exams. I did not react as I would have in the past but, instead, tried to be there as a supportive mother and an open-minded family member.

We asked questions, followed directions, and tried to be informed consumers by learning all we could about the disease and the treatments.

I began to believe that when the physician, the patient, and the family all worked together in unison for the sake of a good outcome, it would be beneficial for everyone. At least I hoped so.

Eventually Adam was put on a mild medication and his ejection fraction went back up to 55%. He continued to have annual echoes, and his results have remained stable.

When he first moved to California to attend school, he would normally return home for his follow up exams, but this year, it was not possible. Due to his schedule and classes, he was unable to arrange it successfully.

During our next conversation, he told me he was going to see his primary care physician to see if she would complete his annual exam and refill his prescription. Evidently, it didn't work out the way he had hoped.

The situation was complicated because his insurance was now through his college and would only cover medical treatments in California. His doctor, understandably, would not give him medications for something she knew nothing about.

In the end, the local office agreed to fax his records to California, and ultimately he was able to get what he needed. But the situation was a stark reminder of the complexity and fragility of the healthcare system and all the time and energy it takes to maneuver through it.

A few years later, Adam was admitted to the hospital through the emergency room for a severe cellulitis.

Although it was commonplace in my work environment, I experienced first-hand how confusing a hospital admission can be.

One by one doctors came to assess him and each would ask the same questions: "How did this happen? When did it start?"

As they left, we would ask each other, "Who was that? Is it orthopedics or infectious disease? Who was here from that group yesterday?"

As a new doctor would arrive each day and discuss his case, we had to keep a log of the names, practice groups, and hospitalists involved in his care. On-call coverage, specialty consults, and large physician and nurse practitioner practices made continuity of care challenging. All were excellent but differed in their diagnostics and treatments so as a family, keeping track of it all was vital.

When he was finally discharged, he was told to follow up with his primary care physician who had to be told the entire scenario as well and given access to the records so he understood the situation clearly.

Adam compared it to the telephone game where you whisper a sentence to multiple people one after another and see how the information is altered as it is repeated at the end.

The days of one medical provider are gone. This shift has positively transformed the quality of our health care but made the patient and family experience more complicated.

As family members, there was anxiety about making sure we understood the information correctly but, as a nurse, I realized I needed to be more pro-active in relieving that anxiety for my patients. Making good decisions is based on clarity of information and we in health care need to be more judicious in assisting in that process.

Walking the tightrope of life is hard enough but add in the emotional turmoil of being sick, multiple physicians, information overload, insurance obstacles, and the medical record complication and you get that familiar stomach-in-the-throat feeling of loss of control—and loss of control is the biggest barrier to our medical relationships.

Chapter 21

Jeff

As I looked around the room, I realized it had been quite a while since I had to spend any time in a hospital waiting room. I walk past one each day at work and direct people to that end of the hallway when they are lost, but I hadn't given much thought to what it is like to be in the midst of it all again until now.

The carpet was stained; the trash cans overflowing with take-out containers and half full drink cups; the hum of conversations filling the room like the buzzing of bees in a garden of spring flowers.

Over the past few years, our lives had changed in ways that were still hard to believe. Jeff and Ellen decided to move to Virginia for employment opportunities, and Adam graduated with his PhD, married his girlfriend Stephanie, and took a job in the Washington DC area. Both boys from the west coast now living in the east!

My sister Jo passed away earlier in the year from the effects of her multiple sclerosis and my first grandchild was born. It seemed the circle of life was a stark reality for my family this year.

There was a tornado warning in place when my phone rang. I almost didn't answer it because I needed to close the windows and move downstairs for safety. Jeff had been on my mind that day because we were in daily contact since the birth of his daughter and he hadn't answered my email yet. I knew he was excited about the World Cup soccer games so I figured he was busy watching them that afternoon.

As I finally came across my phone, I noticed it was Ellen calling. I remembered that she was out of town so I thought she was just touching base as we sometimes do.

"Judi," she said with a tearful voice. "There is something wrong with Jeff. You need to come as soon as you can."

The howling wind and torrential rain outside mimicked the feeling inside me as I learned the details of the situation.

Jeff had not shown up at daycare to pick up his daughter so they called the emergency number which happened to be a neighbor who was also a critical care nurse. As she entered the house, she found Jeff unconscious in a chair with the television on. He had a thready pulse and his breathing was shallow but he was unresponsive. The paramedics had taken him to the ER and this is where he was when I received the call.

I got a flight as soon as I could the next morning while getting updates the whole night through. He woke up from the coma at 1 a.m.; he was confused; they think he had a stroke; they don't know the cause; it may have been carbon monoxide; the house was being tested; MRI ordered. Receiving so much information from 600 miles away was excruciating but not being able to see him when I arrived was worse.

As soon as I entered the building, I headed straight for the ICU. I learned that there were restricted visiting hours in this particular unit and I had a three hour wait before I could see my son. Despite the open visitation policy, I was told it was manager dependent and this manager had set hours.

"She believes families can interfere with care," the clerk told me. It seemed impossible in this current healthcare environment but it was true. So I waited.

So many things go through a person's mind when there is a crisis but not being able to see your loved one intensifies the fear. How did this happen? It seemed so surreal.

I oscillated between panic and tears realizing I may never see my son again. The memories flooded in: our last conversation; how he checked in with me every day; how he teased me about not responding to his emails quickly like I used to do to him.

"Are you there?" I would ask when I didn't hear from him and he would laugh and answer me with some silly line.

The last few months however, had been very busy for me and I was the one not responding in a timely fashion.

Finally I got a text saying "Where are YOU?" As I remembered this, I grabbed my phone and quickly read the message again—was this how our life together was going to end?

At last I was allowed in to see him. Jeff was conscious but very confused and, after a CT scan and lots of blood work, there was still no known cause for his condition. Frustration set in for all of us—MRI had been ordered but not yet done; restricted visiting hours; the neurologist was in another city and wasn't going to see him until the following day.

We were living on borrowed time and no one seemed to be concerned except the family. At least that is how it felt.

Ellen worked for a non-profit medical organization so she began making calls to her physician peers for help. After they arrived, we all sat in the hallway and developed a plan. Colleagues began calling in experts in the field. The hospital system did not like this interference but as uncomfortable as it was, we needed to protect our loved one.

One by one they agreed to look at his films and other tests to see it through another's eyes. They got the MRI moved up to urgent status and, after a few phone calls, the neurologist begrudgingly came back that evening to evaluate Jeff.

What a shame to have to use the system in this way—what if there had been no connective person? We didn't even know what had caused the stroke but we were sure not ready to just give up on the situation.

After all the test results were in, it was determined that Jeff had suffered a bilateral symmetrical thalamic stroke. In other words, the damaged area of his brain was the same on both sides of the thalamus area which controls many functions in the body.

The news was devastating enough but in addition, the neurologist painted a grim picture.

"The damage is done. What is dead is dead. It will not return."

Of course we were shocked and overwhelmed. Jeff was a husband and father and in perfect health. Trying to wrap your emotions around this information while struggling to stay in touch with the reality of it all was too much to bear.

Our hope was dwindling but if the system couldn't help him in the way in which it was designed, then we would use the resources we had to get him what he needed as an individual and a loved one.

Our health care system provides quality care to millions of people but it is a complicated process. Taking control of our own health is vital to the outcomes we desire but if we can't speak for ourselves, then having an advocate is important.

It wasn't that the hospital was a bad one; it had an excellent reputation and the physicians were superb. It's just that Jeff had fallen through the cracks and needed that support.

We agreed to be the voice for him because he couldn't make rational decisions at this time and it helped me to have the support of a team who had his best interest at heart....literally.

Chapter 22
Brother

*A*dam and Stephanie had come down from DC and were involved in Jeff's care from the beginning. Adam and Jeff have always been close but even more so over the last few years. Living in California at the same time brought them together physically and emotionally and now both being on the east coast cemented that brotherly relationship.

Adam was a calming force in this sea of emotions. He talked to Jeff in his normal fashion and never lost patience with him when he was confused. His concern was obvious but he did not let it interfere with their relationship and I saw Jeff look in Adam's direction many times when he was searching for an answer.

Jeff's vision was doubled and blurred and when he tried to look at someone, the eyes were off center, but he always knew what side of the room to look when searching for Adam.

Adam brought Jeff's computer to the hospital and tried to help him watch the soccer games and talked to him about all the things they normally would have discussed if they were at home together. He helped ground Jeff back to his previous life and every once in a while you could see that spark of recognition in Jeff's eyes. The rest of us were so emotionally volatile but Adam stood steadfast at his side.

At one point, they believed Jeff had a dissected vertebral artery that could have caused the stroke. The physician came to the room to discuss this and the further testing he wanted to do. Adam was the only one in the room so he listened to the explanation and even reviewed the films with the doctor on the hospital computer.

When we arrived later, Adam told us that he had taken a picture of the computer screen with his phone so we were able to see it. But in addition, he had hit the record button on his phone while the doctor was talking to be sure he got all the correct information on tape for us to review.

We were so grateful and laughed at his ingenuity but so happy to have had the information first hand. Adam was the buoy for all of us in the rocky emotional waters.

In the evening, Jeff was taken down to the Center for Sight to have a visual assessment and Adam went right along with him. He stayed with him in the room and pushed him back in the wheelchair himself instead of waiting for the transporters.

Ellen, Stephanie, and I were in the room when they returned and Adam gave us a full explanation of what had occurred and the possible treatment options. He was a physical and emotional stabilizing force for Jeff just as Jeff had been for him in California when Adam was a student and needed a support system as well.

I stayed each night with Jeff while the others took care of business at home. This night, Jeff was pretty tired and a little more confused due to the fatigue. I said my goodbyes to Adam and as I was making up my chair bed for the night, Jeff said, "He's a good guy."

"Yes he is," I replied without looking up.

"He's my brother; like my printer-wireless but always connected."

At first I thought he was just confused and rambling his thoughts but as I settled in for the night I realized Jeff had a Brother brand computer printer and it had a wireless connection to his laptop!

"Wireless but always connected," I thought smiling broadly. He was beginning to make sense!

After an angiogram the following day, it was determined that Jeff indeed did not have a dissected vertebral artery so the search for a cause continued.

Next, he had a trans esophageal echocardiogram (TEE) where they placed a probe down the throat and looked at the heart from an internal view. This proved to be the breakthrough we needed as it showed Jeff had a patent foramen ovale (PFO).

This is a small hole in the septum of the heart that just doesn't close up correctly after birth. Many people have this phenomena with no adverse effects throughout their lives but every once in a while, a small clot can cross over and get into the arterial blood flow and go to the brain.

In the scheme of things, this was good because it is fixable and relatively safe unlike having a dissected artery. If we had to choose a cause, this would be it.

We met with a cardiologist who explained the options for repairing this malfunction and we returned to his room feeling better. It is always a good thing to have a clear diagnosis before designing a plan for recovery.

Now we knew. He had been scanned and tested from head to toe and all they could find was a small hole in his heart.

When they initially described what they had found, I felt an immediate but short lived pang of guilt. What if I had done something during my pregnancy that made this happen...what if...what if... I decided again not to waste my energy on the small things I could not control and concentrate on those things that I could.

I reflected back on a time a few weeks ago when I was looking ahead at my calendar. This very week that we were living in at the present moment had so many things penciled in for me to do and accomplish that I had spent an evening trying to figure it all out.

I had no interest in some of the appointments but felt that obligation we all put on ourselves to please others before pleasing ourselves. Now here I was in the middle of this crisis and those things seemed so trivial.

Not that normal life and social and work schedules aren't important... they are, but only when kept in perspective. Jeff had lived a very busy and hectic life before this as well but in this moment none of that matter to him. He wasn't worried about his schedule but about people.

"Where is my mom?" he asked Ellen on the phone as I was standing right next to him. At this moment he did not recognize me but that was okay. I was here with him through it all and somehow that calendar wasn't so important.

Eventually I would follow up with the things I missed and life would go on but in this present moment, I needed to be connected to my son.

Later that night when we were alone, Jeff said, "Mom, can we talk?"

"Sure," I answered quickly. He knew who I was and that I was there, and, after some small talk, he drifted off to sleep.

As I curled up in my chair and prepared for the night, my heart was filled with joy and love. I knew that this is exactly where I wanted to be no matter the date or event penciled in on a day timer.

Chapter 23
Of House and Home

"**D**o you want to go home today or tomorrow?" the doctor asked as he made his rounds.

"Today!" Jeff and I said in harmony.

It had not been a good hospital stay and we just wanted to get him home and under our care. We made all the calls and by 3 p.m., Jeff was discharged.

It wasn't that the staff was negligent; the care was just fragmented. Information wasn't passed on from shift to shift; communication between doctors and bedside staff was disjointed; no real case management or discharge instructions to know what steps to take once we took him home.

We weren't even sure who was in charge of his care since he had several specialists, but we decided that we would just get him home and then figure out a plan.

I recalled some of my former patients and all the emotional turmoil that was evident in many of their family members. They wanted to go home but had so many questions about that process.

Fear of the unknown and change in the life they previously knew often expressed itself in frustration with me and many times I didn't have all the answers. I now realized what a daunting task it was for them and vowed to be more cagniscent of follow-up instructions and information for loved ones. I was now that person living that same experience. The conflict was apparent.

Being a nurse, I realized how important it was to be in familiar surroundings. Many times a patient's confusion is dissipated when they get back to their normal living space and we were hoping this was the case for Jeff. Also, Jeff had not seen his daughter since his hospitalization and he missed her terribly.

Watching Jeff interact with his family in their home was the best lesson of all. As I observed Ellen assisting Jeff when he needed it while maintaining his dignity and self-image, I realized this was better than any medication he could ever be prescribed. Being with his family in their private living quarters and feeling the love between them was the miracle we were all meant to experience when we were put on this earth.

I remembered back to when they had moved from California last year. I was the one upset because I loved everything about that area. The house, the weather, the retail areas; everything was so perfect.

I had so many wonderful visits with Jeff and Adam and saw such beautiful landscapes; I almost went into withdrawal when I heard they were moving. Could they ever live this perfect life on the east coast?

Even when they settled into their rental home and I had visited a few times, I thought back to those California days and felt sadness for that life I believed they left behind. But here we were, and it seemed the perfect place and the perfect life with the perfect people.

Several of their friends stopped by that day to see Jeff and offer support. We all spent the night at the house with them and slept on air mattresses and the couch but no one seemed to care. The point was we were all together sharing in the good and not so good things. No matter the temperature or zip code, Jeff was finally back where he belonged—home.

We should all be so fortunate to find a place so exquisite and beautiful in which to dwell and built by the healing force of love.

The following day was Father's Day and we were still living in the chaotic process of adjusting to Jeff having a stroke. We wanted to do something to celebrate it but no one had their act together enough to figure it out.

Then Cheryl appeared at the door like Roma Downey Jr. in "Touched by an Angel."

"Would you like to come over for a Father's Day brunch?" she asked in her quiet sweet way. It was an answer to our dilemma.

Cheryl was the neighbor who had found Jeff unconscious and called 911 just a few days ago. Her family and Jeff and Ellen had become fast friends so she was the contact person they listed for the day care. Now here she was rescuing us from ourselves and giving us back some sense of normalcy. Who says angels don't walk the earth!

As we sat around the table and shared laughter and great food, I felt my granddaughter's gum and found her first tooth had come through! Everyone celebrated this occurrence together telling Jeff that was his Father's Day gift, and I saw the smile come back to his face.

I stood back in the room and just looked at what was going on here. It was much more than a brunch to celebrate a day out of the year or a tooth that had come through. It was the power of friends using food and fellowship to celebrate life with all its brokenness and flaws. It was a way to take the yearning to help that we all feel when we want to be of assistance to another human being but don't know how or what to do.

Food and fellowship are the vehicles used to transport the love and caring we want to express but don't know how to do it in an acceptable way. Like insulin transports glucose through the membrane to nourish the cells, food and fellowship carry the need to help to those who need to receive it.

As the days progressed, I witnessed this time and time again. Each day, someone stopped by to drop off food to nourish our bodies and fellowship to nourish our souls. Their friends actually made up an excel spread sheet for each day of the week and everyone signed up for a day of food so we never had to worry about what to eat. We had access to the spreadsheet so we even knew what was coming each day!

One by one they came and brought food and you could see in their eyes that they were getting as much if not more out of this than we were. The power of giving nourishment to others is an innate trait in each of us and even though Jeff having a stroke is a horrible way to manifest the good in others; that is exactly what it did.

As a nurse, I watch visitors as they bring food items in for my patients because they want to nourish their loved one, and as a family member, my first question was always "Are you eating okay?" After each chemotherapy treatment, my sister and I would go out to dinner that evening and out for breakfast again the following morning. When we don't know what to do for those we love, we feed.

Food is what we use to represent the hope and love we want to share with others whether it be a social event or an illness. We all have the need to sustain and nurture our souls as well as our bodies and food can be the catalyst for this phenomenon.

Being a mother and a nurse, I have the opportunity to observe this not only with Jeff and his friends but also in my work. I can nourish my patients not just with food but with the care and knowledge of my profession. Just as a meal excel spreadsheet demonstrates the love of others for Jeff, I have the privilege of nourishing others back to health. I am honored to be able to be a part of both.

Chapter 24
Change is Coming

"Letting go" is a term used in various situations, but I never thought I would have to let go of one of my children. Jeff was forced to let go of who he was through a brain injury over which he had no control and we now had to learn who the new Jeff might become.

Pre-stroke Jeff was very left brained; data, science, and facts controlled his belief system but after the stroke, we witnessed a different right brained personality.

Going to the Edgar Cayce Health Center to get a massage and stroll through the library to look for books on the body mind spirit connection would not have been of interest to Jeff a few weeks ago but here we were enjoying that moment with him.

"Maybe there is something here that can help me," he said as we arrived.

In some ways, it is so confusing. When I cried, I said I want my son back but yet I looked at him and I still see the same physical Jeff.

What was it I wanted back? A personality? I am not sure what I was grieving for…Jeff the way I knew and loved him I guess. But then

I think this was teaching us all such a big lesson in life; holding on to what was might hinder what greater things lie ahead.

As hard as it might be, letting go might be a gift in disguise. Don't get me wrong, I am not saying I can do this, but every once in a while I got a glimpse of the big picture here through Jeff's eyes.

It was very sad to see him struggle to type one word on his computer because he could not see, but he didn't give up. He sat for long periods of time trying to just type his name and it was only a short time ago he was remoting in to my home computer to help me fix a problem. If he could let go, why couldn't I?

Every once in a while he called himself "dumb and slow" but it never stopped him from trying to grow into who he was becoming. I thought there was something bigger than we knew here and I was just trying to figure it all out.

We went to appointment after appointment and he listened and tried to learn everything he could at each one of them. We went to physical therapy and he tried desperately to do the balance exercises and then turned around and smiled at us when he accomplished them.

He thanked me for watching out for him on the escalators at the mall when we spent the day together and asked me if I was lonely living by myself.

"I don't want you to be alone," he said. At the end of each day he goes to bed exhausted but relatively content.

At physical therapy one day, I had to leave because it was just so emotionally difficult to witness. On the way home, he asked me why I got up and left. I made an excuse about finding my phone but he knew better.

"Is it because it is too hard to watch?" he asked.

"Yes," I said.

"I remember feeling that way when I came home from college and seeing you," he replied.

"I wasn't sick then."

"I know," he said, "but you were very sad after Rob died and I couldn't stand to see you that way."

I had no idea he had ever felt that and he had never shared that before. So what was it that I wanted to fix or get back?

What I learned from this experience with Jeff is that he, just like my patients, had no choice but to let go of life as he knew it, but I do have a choice.

I watched and learned how he adjusted and modified things he used to know in order to learn a new way. Just as many of my patients do after a diagnosis or a life altering event, he took the reality of the situation and used it to prioritize the future without all the scars from the past.

Maybe I could start to do the same in my personal and work life and get out of the way of myself to become who I really am without all the attachments and expectations and emotional reactions. If he can do it and if they can do it, at least I can try.

Conclusion

I have been a semi runner most of my adult life. As I was out for a run one evening, I was looking for a route that was long enough for my training schedule that day. I found myself in a nearby condo development that had pathways running all through it, and as I progressed, the path led me to a steep hill.

I was tired and really did not want to continue. I mentally reviewed every excuse why I should turn around and go back, and I griped about the hill being part of the running path.

"Why would they put this big hill right in the middle of a walking trail? "Who designed this anyway?"

For reasons I cannot explain, however, I proceeded up the hill. I was huffing and puffing as I reached the top, wondering what the heck I was going to encounter when I got there.

"Probably another hill," I said out loud in a sarcastic tone.

But what I found took me completely by surprise and opened my eyes to something I would have never imagined. The most spectacular panoramic view appeared in front of me as I glanced up at the open area before me.

The winding river with boats that looked like tiny specks on the glassy surface; a view of the city's buildings and skyscrapers that I had never seen before; a clear royal blue sky, and chattering birds flying back and forth among the multitude of flowering trees that lined the crest of the hill. It was one of the most stunning sights I had ever encountered, and I sat on the bench atop the hill and took it all in.

I realized that if I had stuck with my original perception and expectations of the hill and not faced it head on, I would have never had the experience of a beautiful and positive outcome.

The same thing applies to our medical relationships. There is no "how-to guide" in our patient admission packets, and most nurses don't get healthcare communication courses in their rigorous training so we learn through our trial and error experiences.

It took me a long time to take what I had learned from my medical experiences and use them to teach others not to make the same assumptions as I did in similar situations. I even tried to keep a sense of humor about it all.

On one of my trips to California, some of Jeff's friends invited us to share their box seats at a professional soccer game. As time progressed, their four year old was getting restless and lost interest in the game so I was trying to entertain her to no avail. Without even thinking, I reached up and pulled off my wig exposing my bare head.

"Look Emma," I said. I can take off my hair!" Emma was astounded to say the least.

She laughed and said over and over, "Do it again!"

The mood of the entire room changed in one single moment. Emma was happy and the rest of the group could relax about what to say and not say to me. I was just another person in the room who happened to have no hair.

Not taking myself so seriously helped me and the others to have an open conversation about my current situation. Being able to talk about it without all the baggage of the illness opened up a dialogue that was beneficial to all of us. It cultivated the bridge to a friendship that still remains today.

Our connection to each other is the key, and if we just react as we always have in the past, there is no opportunity to change the future of our healthcare relationships.

My mom used to say, "If you always do what you've always done, then you'll always get what you've always gotten." She was smarter than I thought.

Fast forward to present day. Adam's last ejection fraction was 55% and he continues to live a purpose driven life. Jeff got cleared to drive again and is now working a full time job. I am still the manager of the cardiac unit, and I have just past my fifth annual post cancer checkup with flying colors.

I wish I could say that I have completely transformed my thinking and reactions to patients and families when they are unkind to the hospital staff and remember that they have a history I know nothing about.

I wish I could say I never refer to patients as a room number or a diagnosis.

I wish I could say that all nurses communicate with patients and their families in an open and understanding way all of the time, and that patients and families appreciate and comprehend the complexity of the nurses' multifaceted role in their care.

Instead, I say it is a confused and perplexing state where everyone is just trying to do his or her best. I have witnessed a patient complimenting the staff for a certain action while at the very same time another one wants to report them for doing the exact same thing.

Having been in each situation, I believe it is a matter of perception of the circumstances and a lack of understanding of the position of the other person. And fear. And control. Or the lack of it. Or a combination of all of them. The conflict of caring.

Many medical institutions have begun to develop policies and committees directed at incorporating the nurse, the family, and the patient all together into the healthcare experience, but until it is brought down to the grass roots level, it will not succeed. It is like building a house from the rooftop down.

Instead, going to the foundation of the experience is essential for any change to occur. The one on one, human being to human being experience where change and understanding of the situations takes place. Hopefully telling stories like mine will be the catalyst for that change.

When my patient was upset that I was discussing my life instead of attending to his, he did not care what the policy said. Instead, he cared what I said directly to him.

When I was upset that my nurse was going to lunch when I might have cancer in my lymph nodes, I did not care that we had a committee addressing those very issues. I cared what she said to me in that encounter at that minute in my personal experience.

It is not that those policies aren't important, but until each individual understands the position and experience of the other person at that moment, they are but words on paper.

Patients are bombarded with information through the news media, and nurses are regulated by numerous governing bodies. All of these were established with good intentions, but in the process, we have lost some of that human connection that is essential to healing.

In times of stress, it is difficult to pull back and look at that whole big picture and try to understand the perspective of others. But if we are going to work together as one human being caring about another, we have to listen and understand the viewpoint of others and approach our healthcare experience with that in hand.

That Rocky Mountain view is so much better than the piece of rock; tightrope walking is easier when there is a net to break a fall; penguins fight to the end for the sake of their eggs; the view at the top of the hill is better than the one from below.

No matter what the metaphor of life may be, the message is always the same: Instead of reacting to those individual situations as in the past, it is better to take the time to step back and listen and learn and remember and think and talk and share and communicate and ….just remove those barriers that cause conflict and simply take care of each other, for goodness sake.

Made in the USA
Charleston, SC
21 September 2013

Made in the USA
Middletown, DE
11 May 2019